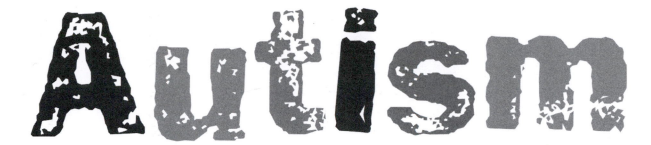

Autism

A social skills approach for children and adolescents

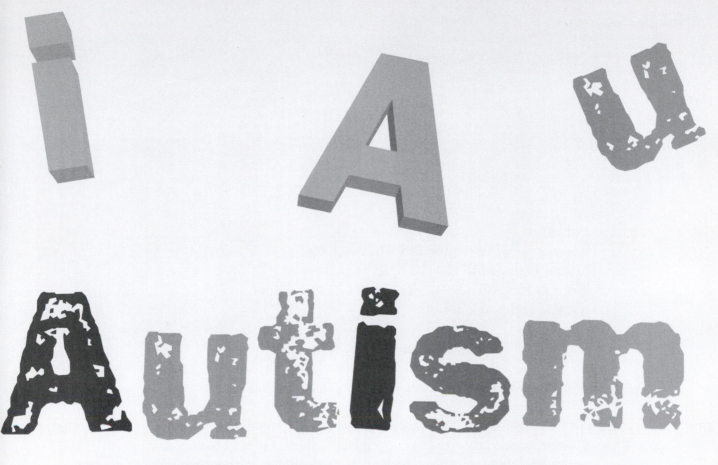

Autism

A social skills approach for children and adolescents

**Maureen Aarons
& Tessa Gittens**

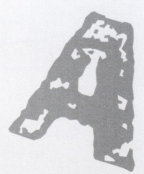

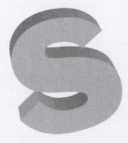

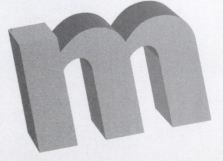

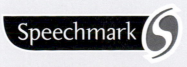

Speechmark

www.speechmark.net

Published by
Speechmark Publishing Ltd, 70 Alston Drive, Bradwell Abbey,
Milton Keynes MK13 9HG, UK
Tel: +44 (0)1908 326944   Fax: +44 (0)1908 326960
www.speechmark.net

002-3088/Printed in the United Kingdom/4020

British Library Cataloguing in Publication Data
Aarons, Maureen
    Autism: a social skills approach for children and adolescents
    1. Autism   2. Autistic children   3. Autistic youth
    I. Title   II. Gittens, Tessa
    618.9'2'8982

ISBN: 978 086388 319 4

Contents

Acknowledgements

We are indebted to the adults with autism who have shared their experiences so openly with us, especially Therese Jolliffe, and to the children who have participated in our groups and given us insights and understanding as well as much enjoyment.

Preface

Although we use the term 'parents', we wish to make it clear that the term includes single parents, carers or, indeed, anyone who is acting *in loco parentis*.

Please note that, for consistency of style, the pronoun 'he' is generally used throughout the book when referring to the child with autism. The choice of the masculine pronoun was influenced by the higher incidence of autism in males.

Inevitably, some of the organizations and procedures referred to in the text may not be available or practised outside the United Kingdom. It is not possible to provide information about facilities and legislation in other countries, and we have to assume that readers will be able to locate for themselves what is relevant to the needs of particular children. Similarly, we refer to songs and rhymes that are part of British culture. Again, we assume that readers can substitute their own choices and preferences as necessary.

MAUREEN AARONS

TESSA GITTENS

Introduction

Autism is now known to be a cognitive disorder, with neurobiological associations, affecting all aspects of social development. As speech and language therapists, working in both the community and educational settings, over a considerable period of time, we are in a position to relate our everyday experiences to the research findings that have burgeoned in recent years. These findings underpin our approach to remediation, which is that a disorder affecting social functioning should be remediated through approaches which focus on social functioning. Since social disability is the essence of autism, it would seem misguided to focus on peripheral deficits which exist in many individuals with autism, but are not by any means central to the disorder. This is why programmes such as auditory integration training, sensory integration therapy and behaviour modification techniques, as well as some of the well publicized alternative approaches, will not be effective in the long term. Although many of these procedures may have an immediate appeal because they seem to have something very tangible to offer in the here and now, they do not address the underlying disability. We would argue that progress may be made, however, in the natural history of the disorder; some progress takes place anyway! It must be accepted that there are no short cuts to remediation. It is a slow, painstaking process, but much can be achieved when children with autism have access to a social skills programme, preferably within an appropriate educational setting.

The aim of this book is to present practical ideas that will form the basis for programmes of intervention for children with autism. At the outset, we need to make it clear that the content is aimed at children with normal or near normal cognitive abilities, rather than those whose autism accompanies severe learning disability. However, those using the book will be able to ascertain for themselves what is appropriate or what can be adapted to suit the needs of less able children.

Many books are available which describe the history of the condition of autism, and it is not necessary for us to reiterate what has already been well documented. Nevertheless, it must be acknowledged that intervention strategies reflect changing ideas and levels of knowledge about the causes and nature of the disorder. It is therefore necessary to refer to this legacy in the light of current research and what is now regarded as good practice.

Until very recently, it was usual to refer to 'autistic' children (or adults), which supported the idea that individuals with this disorder were all the same. Checklists of so-called features were used for diagnosis, and this reinforced the notion of a discrete and uniform condition. Little wonder that there were endless arguments about whether a child was, or was not, autistic on this basis. It is human nature to categorize and classify, and those children deemed *not* to be autistic were often trailed from one specialist centre to another, picking up an assortment of diagnostic labels, while their real needs went unrecognized. Readers may be familiar with such terms as 'High Level Language Disorder', 'Aphasia', 'Attention Deficit Disorder' and 'Semantic–Pragmatic Disorder', among others, all of which reflect perhaps a single aspect of the much wider disorder of autism. We now refer to children or individuals 'with autism', which supports the notion of variability, and the concept of a *continuum* of severity. The term 'Asperger Syndrome' is now widely used to describe able individuals whose abilities place them at the upper end of the autistic continuum.

In order to accommodate the variability of autism, with the supposition that sub-groups may be identified within the diagnostic framework, some professionals promote the use of the term 'Autistic Spectrum Disorder'. This term may well prevail in the future as acceptance of an autism phenotype with as yet no precise boundaries gains favour over traditional diagnostic criteria which may no longer be considered useful. The notion of an 'autism phenotype' will make sense to those professionals working with the families of children with autism, who see in family members subtle social deficits typical of autism, but without the obvious and disabling features which present in the affected child.

Dr Lorna Wing (1979) enabled us to move away from rigid checklists by pinpointing the particular areas of difficulty that are specific to autism. They affect social functioning and are known as 'the Triad of Social Impairments'. These impairments affect relationships, communication and understanding/imagination. To identify autism, we need to recognize whether an individual has qualitative difficulties in these areas. This is far removed from diagnosing on the basis of whether or not a child cuddles his mother or maintains eye contact! The concept of the Triad is a complex one encompassing gradations of impairment, and these impairments can be very subtle indeed, especially in more able individuals.

In the 1940s, Leo Kanner (1943) first identified the condition of autism and listed a number of core features which were necessary for a diagnosis. Perhaps this is the reason why, some 50 years later, diagnosis is still often linked to checklists that reflect a medical model approach, despite the fact that the only tried and tested treatment of the condition is appropriate education and management. It is as true now as in Kanner's day that children with autism not only look normal but are often particularly attractive. Not surprisingly, this encouraged Kanner to presume that they were invariably intelligent, especially as they often displayed a range of particular skills in some developmental areas. As an explanation for the children's apparent withdrawal and social isolation, Kanner believed that poor parenting was the cause of the condition. The mother was almost invariably blamed, and the term 'refrigerator mother' was most unfairly applied. With this level of understanding, treatment for autism was based on attempts to remediate relationships between mother and child, with the supposition that, once this had been achieved, the child would develop normally. Foremost among these approaches was 'Holding Therapy', which like many other unsubstantiated remedies became popular for a while. The notion of autism as an emotional disorder became discredited as knowledge about the biological nature of the condition increased. However, despite evidence to refute this simplistic explanation for the generation of autism, centres still exist where this opinion is supported. Although family dynamics most certainly play a part in the overall picture of children with autism, there is no evidence to suggest that they are the cause of the condition. It is a fact that good or unsatisfactory parenting will have an effect on all children in any family, including those who have autism.

The term 'Asperger Syndrome', relates to the children who were described in 1944 as having 'an autistic psychopathy' by Hans Asperger (see Frith, 1991) whose writings, which focused particularly on behaviour, appeared at about the same time as Kanner's. The behaviour problems often displayed by children with autism subsequently encouraged the development of behaviour modification approaches to remediation. Once again, the focus was based on an aspect of the condition, without an appreciation or understanding of the whole picture.

Recently, there has been an upsurge of interest in the behaviour modification methods of Lovaas (1996), which were originally pioneered in the 1960s. His methods have been modified to provide parents with a package of intervention which enables them to feel actively involved in their child's development. Although the effectiveness of this approach in relation to social development and communication is questionable, it may be of use in reducing severe behaviour problems.

Over the years, attention has centred on other aspects of anomalous development. There is considerable evidence that many individuals with autism have unusual, if not extreme, responses to sensory stimulation. These anomalies have been the focus of the development of remediation programmes such as 'Sensory Integration Therapy' (King, 1991) and 'Auditory Integration Training' (Rimland & Edelson, 1995). Since difficulties with sensory functioning are not evident in all people with autism, they cannot be regarded as a criterion for diagnosis. However, sensory dysfunction should be taken into account as a feature frequently associated with the condition that may require attention.

Although education has proved to be the most effective approach in the treatment of autism, here too inappropriate assumptions were made, based on misunderstandings about the condition. There was a belief that an intensive education programme would break through the barrier of autism and allow a normal child to emerge. Rote learning and islets of ability were mistaken for knowledge and understanding, and consequently expectations of outcome were unrealistic and misconceived.

Abnormalities of language have always been regarded as fundamental to the condition of autism. Speech and language therapists are often among the first professionals to see young children with autism, and have had to bear the burden of a widely held belief that, if only the child could talk, all would be well. In this frame of reference, cognitive difficulties and behaviour problems are marginalized, and seen as unconnected to what is perceived solely as a language disorder. The use of the label 'Semantic–Pragmatic Disorder', first emerging in the 1980s (Bishop, 1989) as a diagnostic term, typified this misunderstanding. It was only when evident social impairments were understood as intrinsic to the condition, and not a consequence, that children with these difficulties in the *use* of language could be more accurately diagnosed as having autism. As a corollary to the confusion about the use of language, there was also a belief that the introduction of a manual sign system would bypass the lack of spoken language. This was a naive assumption that did not take into account the wide-ranging nature of autism, which affects all modes of communication, both verbal and non-verbal. However, manual sign systems do have a place in teaching programmes. Non-verbal children may benefit from being taught some basic signs to make their needs known. For more able children, signs may enhance understanding of specific concepts — for example, prepositions and pronouns.

Advocates of 'Facilitated Communication' (Biklen, 1993) held the same naive convictions, ignoring scientific evidence in favour of unsubstantiated beliefs in a practice which had more in common with religious fervour than an actual understanding of autism. Sadly, many professionals and parents continue to be misled and there have been a number of cases where abuse was alleged by well-meaning but misguided facilitators.

We have already mentioned the variability of autism and that it can co-exist with learning disability and sensory anomalies. However, the picture is rather more complex than this. Not only will children with autism have varying patterns of development, but they will also exhibit considerable variations between one another. In addition, there may be links to other conditions known to occur in conjunction with autism. Fragile-X Syndrome, Tuberous Sclerosis and Rett's

Syndrome, for example, have long been associated, and more recently Tourette Syndrome has been added to the list.

When Uta Frith's book, *Autism: Explaining The Enigma*, was published in 1989, the impact on remediation programmes was considerable. She described the cognitive impairments inherent in autism that made sense of Wing's Triad. Frith's work on theory of mind and central coherence encapsulated the essence of the difficulties experienced by children with autism and pointed the way to relevant approaches to teaching and intervention. Deficits in theory of mind are shown by the inability of children with autism to understand other people's ideas, thoughts and feelings. In other words, they cannot 'mind read'. Problems with central coherence result in the child having difficulty in knowing what to attend to and extracting what is meaningful. Simon Baron-Cohen (1995) and Fran Happe (1994) have since made a considerable contribution to our understanding of both theory of mind and central coherence in relation to autism. (*See Chapter 1*.)

Another core deficit at the psychological level described in the literature is the failure to develop normal 'executive function' (Ozonoff *et al*, 1994), which relates to people with autism having problems in planning and organization. These difficulties are believed to underlie the repetitive and perseverative behaviours seen in many individuals with the condition. (A possible alternative explanation for these behaviours is suggested in Chapter 4.) It is open to debate whether 'executive function' should be considered as a separate deficit in relation to organization and planning. It could be argued that an impaired ability to extract what is meaningful, that is, difficulties with central coherence, would directly affect the individual's ability to plan and organize. In other words, central coherence underpins executive function.

It is important that those involved in the care and/or teaching of children with autism should keep abreast of research developments, so that their intervention and management are based on ideas which reflect consolidated knowledge about the condition, rather than claims which have not been validated. It may be difficult for therapists, teachers and psychologists, as well as parents, to judge which research has something to offer them, and it is very easy to be demoralized by jargon and convoluted academic language; it is our view that practical experience provides them with a yardstick to judge the value of new theories and recognize those which enhance their understanding of the children with autism with whom they have contact. Our own understanding of autism was undoubtedly enhanced by the revelation of theory of mind and central coherence, which made sense of so much and enabled us to develop new ideas.

Any practitioner carrying out an intervention programme has a responsibility not to present it as a panacea. Autism is a developmental disability and does not go away. At best, appropriate intervention enables individuals with autism to make the most of their capabilities and develop strategies to cope with their deficits. However, this may be difficult for parents to accept: they will almost always look for a cure, and this is entirely understandable. It is very easy for the experienced professional to feel exasperation when parents seem to waste time and money on unsubstantiated 'remedies' because they 'cannot bear to leave any stone unturned'. The practitioner must not take this personally; many people need to find things out for themselves, and no amount of advice will deflect them from their quest. Ultimately, the majority of parents subscribe to approaches that make sense, rather than those based on wishful thinking.

It was the work of Wendy Rinaldi (1992, 1994) which drew our attention to the relevance of social skills training for children with autism. She developed her 'Social Use of Language Programme' with other client groups in mind, without being aware of its applicability to children whose fundamental disability was social impairment. For this we owe her a real debt, as it enabled us to develop a better understanding of the needs of these children and the ways in which we could intervene to enhance their social functioning.

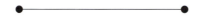

A checklist is provided for easy reference where appropriate at the end of each chapter. In addition, at the end of the book, appendices include model letters and forms, useful addresses and suggestions for books and equipment.

CHAPTER

1 Assessment

Since autism was first identified there has been a considerable amount of research into various aspects of the condition. A review of this research (Bailey *et al*, 1996) describes the current state of knowledge and highlights the need to develop an integrated approach to the evaluation of research findings. These include genetic, neuropsychological and neurobiological perspectives and reference is made to the apparent increase in the incidence of autism. This could be at least partly explained by the extension of diagnostic boundaries to include individuals who do not conform to traditional diagnostic criteria while clearly displaying the social deficits inherent in autism. As practitioners we have observed subtle social anomalies in the families of children with autism, affecting one or other parent, usually the father, as well as siblings. Bailey *et al*'s paper, which refers to 'a phenotype' for autistic spectrum disorders, provides 'respectability' to observations by those working in the field that autism is by no means a rare condition.

In other words, elements of autism are indeed widespread. For a multitude of reasons, society now demands explanations, and provision for any child who fails to develop according to expectations, and we can now identify clusters of developmental problems, which previously would have been ignored or explained away. It is our view that, if autism causes the child to experience problems which impinge on family life and educational progress as well as social competence, diagnosis is vital. We have personal acquaintance with academically gifted adults with autism, who describe lives fraught with difficulties and unhappiness, and for whom a diagnosis, although made when they were in their twenties, brought feelings of considerable relief.

There are two uses for assessment: one is for diagnostic purposes and the other as a starting point for intervention. Intervention can apply to both teaching and therapy, and there is no necessity to draw distinctions between one and the other. Some users of this book may be working with children who have received a formal diagnosis of autism, while others may suspect its presence in children with a range of different diagnostic labels, some of which we referred to in the Introduction. This really does not matter. What does matter is the recognition of the child's profile of impairments, both social and cognitive, which are evident in the areas of the Triad (*see page 2*). In other words, the question to be addressed is: *Does this child's range of difficulties make sense in the context of autism?* If this is the case, there should be no need to become embroiled in arguments about the merits of one label rather than another. Assessment should address a child's individual needs, and must be wide-ranging to encompass the variations and seeming paradoxes which are inherent in the condition. It is very easy to focus on, and be misled by, islets of ability, as well as particular areas of developmental difficulty, such as dyspraxia.

Because children with autism are so variable, the process of assessment can be likened to the completion of a jigsaw as, piece by piece, the disparate aspects of the child's skills and deficits are combined to construct a meaningful picture. The face of a child imposed on a single jigsaw piece makes an evocative and apposite logo for the UK National Autistic Society. It is important to remember that, in the natural history of the condition of autism, changes occur as children mature. Many of the overt features of autism may recede, so that by middle childhood the picture may be very different from that of early infancy. Autism does not go away, but presents in a variety of ways at different stages in a child's development. Because the picture does not stay the same, it is not at all unusual for a professional to meet an older child with behaviour and communication difficulties, and fail to notice the underlying social impairments. Assumptions are made on the basis of current problems without reference to the child's early history, which may hold all the diagnostic evidence. A snapshot view is always unsatisfactory. Assessment must extend beyond a clinical setting, to include extended observations of the child's social functioning in real-life situations.

Our publication, *The Autistic Continuum* (1992), provides a detailed and structured assessment schedule, which readers may wish to refer to, since it is not our intention to replicate in this book what has already been explained. However, we do need to highlight the essential aspects of assessment in order to ensure that intervention is relevant and realistic.

Where should assessment begin? The simple answer is: at the very beginning. The pregnancy of the mother and the birth history may provide information which is relevant. Brain damage may have occurred; there may have been infections and a subsequent range of illnesses and developmental difficulties, any of which may point to learning disability in conjunction with autism. Because autism has a known genetic component, information about the family is relevant, not least because it may have implications for future pregnancies. Siblings and close relatives of individuals with autism are known to have a higher than average incidence of cognitive difficulties that include language delay and dyslexia, as well as different manifestations of autism, or autistic-like behaviour (Bailey *et al*, 1996).

A detailed developmental history is essential, with particular reference to the child's early social development, rather than physical milestones. The latter are often normal or even precocious in children with severe disabilities. Anyone with experience of socially normal babies and young children will be able to identify those who appear self-contained and uninterested in initiating social interaction. Such children may be responsive, especially to rough-and-tumble play and physical input from others, but this can mask their underlying social impairments. These are the babies that fail to engage eye contact or initiate conversations without words, who do not make efforts to share interests and whose only attempts at communication are for their own needs. Research (Baron-Cohen, 1992) has shown that these early indicators of a lack of social reciprocity can indeed be precursors of the condition of autism. The Checklist for Autism in Toddlers (the CHAT) devised by Simon Baron-Cohen (*see page 81*) has proved to be a useful instrument for detecting children who are at risk, as early as age 18 months.

CHAT consists of two sections. Section A is a series of nine simple questions requiring 'yes/no' answers from parents. Section B records observations by the family doctor or health visitor on the occasion of a developmental assessment. Section A is designed to pinpoint whether the child demonstrates joint-attention behaviour (which encompasses the sharing of interests with another person and requesting by pointing) as well as pretend play. Section B records the child's responses to requests that have a social component. To be at risk, a child has to lack both pretend play and joint attention at age 18 months. (*See Appendix, page 81.*)

The attractive appearance of young children with autism is legendary and defies explanation. This makes it all the more difficult for parents to acknowledge the presence of a serious developmental disability. Careful observation at the outset of assessment should reveal the significance of certain anomalous behaviours which, until then, had perhaps not been appreciated. These behaviours may include grimacing, body spinning, hand flapping, repetitive and meaningless activity, unusual and/or dominating interests, a lack of eye contact, and so on. This is not to say that autism should necessarily be diagnosed because of the presence of particular characteristics of the condition. Many children with autism show facets of behaviour which are considerably more subtle. For example, they may relate well to adults in a one to one situation, but do not know how to participate in social play with other children.

Assessment of a child's level of attention is of crucial importance. Typically, children with autism will have only fleeting attention control for anything other than their own choice of activity. Until a child is able to attend to an adult's choice of activity, even if it is only for a very short time, he will not be ready to learn. This is where direct intervention may begin. The aim is to enable a child to develop to a stage of integrated attention which is well controlled and sustained.

It is not at all uncommon for children with autism to exhibit sensory dysfunction. The term 'sensory defensiveness' is sometimes used to describe these difficulties, especially in more able children, and indeed may have been the focus for diagnostic investigation, while the social disabilities have been set aside. The most common sensory abnormalities affect visual and auditory perception, but some children like to touch and smell inappropriately. The prevalence of tiptoe walking among children with autism has been associated with extreme sensitivity in the feet, but there could be other explanations.

Many people, including professionals, are not fully aware of the complexities of play. Parents and carers may well report that the child with autism plays very well when, in reality, all he does is line up cars or engage in repetitive routines with *Lego*®. Similarly, the notion of 'creative play' is not fully understood, and it is easy to interpret derived or learnt play sequences as evidence of creativity. The casual onlooker may well be beguiled by this, but further observation will show that the play does not develop or lead anywhere, and is an end in itself. It is not the presence or absence of play which is significant in children with autism, but its *quality*.

Social play is not beyond many children with autism, and they may enjoy being in the company of other children. However, the sort of games in which they can participate will either be rough-and-tumble play, running about and chasing, or, in the case of older children, board or computer games with clearly defined rules. Play which involves the understanding of subtle social rules is a particular area of difficulty: they do not know how to join in and will often use inappropriate strategies, which may include aggression.

We have already mentioned 'theory of mind', in relation to the work of Uta Frith. She and other researchers use the term 'mentalizing' to describe the ability to understand the thoughts, feelings and intentions of others which is deficient in individuals with autism. However, deficits in mentalizing cannot explain all aspects of autism, and Frith suggests that weak 'central coherence' may explain some of them. This term describes the cognitive process whereby information is extracted to provide meaningful and coherent ideas to make sense of the world. Because children with autism lack 'central coherence', their cognitive difficulties are manifold. The predicament of the person with autism has been likened to that of an alien, or someone from another planet. The only means they have for making sense of the world is their intellectual capability, which may explain why those with autism and learning disability make so little progress. So much information about the world is absorbed without any conscious effort or awareness; knowledge can be applied flexibly to accommodate changing situations and new experiences, and this is what the individual with autism has great difficulty in doing. An indication of these wide-ranging difficulties which govern their lives can be extrapolated by their evident problems with picture sequences. In her book, *Autism: An Introduction to Psychological Theory* (1994), Fran Happe explains with clarity the type of stories which are particularly difficult for them to understand. These involve the process of mentalizing, and only make sense if other people's states of mind are appreciated.

The following example requires an understanding of irony.

> Ann's mother has spent a long time cooking Ann's favourite meal, fish and chips, but when she brings it in to Ann, she is watching TV, and she doesn't even look up, or say thank you. Ann's mother is cross and says, "Well that's very nice, isn't it! That's what I call politeness!"

Is it true what Ann's mother says?
Why does Ann's mother say this?

The next story requires an understanding of white lies.

> Helen waited all year for Christmas because she knew that at Christmas she could ask her parents for a rabbit. Helen wanted a rabbit more than anything in the world. At last Christmas Day arrived and Helen ran to unwrap the big box her parents had given her. She felt sure it would contain a little rabbit in a cage. But when she opened it, with all the family standing round, she found her present was just a boring old set of encyclopaedias, which Helen did not want at all! Still, when Helen's parents asked her how she liked her present, she said, "It's lovely, thank you. It's just what I wanted."

Is it true what Helen said?
Why did she say that to her parents?

All the stories included in the book will be useful for assessing older and more able children with autism. In addition, pictures, cartoons and newspaper cuttings can be used, not only to highlight their difficulties, but as useful materials to enhance understanding.

Psychometric assessment is as relevant to children with autism as to any other diagnostic group, yet this is often put aside during the assessment process, while presenting symptoms are seen as indicators for intervention. For example, a child without language may be expected to respond to intensive speech and language therapy, regardless of the fact that, developmentally, he is at a pre-linguistic stage. In other words, it does not make sense to approach teaching or therapy without reference to the level of cognitive development. If a child's major problems centre around severe learning disability, this should be the focus for management and subsequent educational placement. The presence of autism should then be seen as an additional impairment, not the primary one, and it is important that this is made clear to parents.

The majority of schools for children with severe learning disabilities are now very well aware of the needs of those with autism, and have the expertise to enable such children to make maximum progress.

It is understandable that, when low-functioning children are given a diagnosis, their parents prefer the label 'autism', to 'mental handicap' or 'learning disability'. It enables them to set aside the cognitive deficits in favour of a condition which has an aura of mystery about it, and might even include hope for a cure, however unrealistic. While we accept that there is a real distinction between learning disabled children with autism and those without this additional impairment, the distinction is not as great as that between low- and high-functioning children with autism. It is when children have autism with good cognitive skills that the social impairments must be addressed, as they will inevitably affect educational progress.

Children with autism have problems with all forms of communication. In terms of spoken language, this may range from a complete absence of or interest in communicating to subtle difficulties affecting the use of language. Because children with autism will often produce quite sophisticated utterances with complex syntax, incorrect assumptions are made about their understanding of language. Research has indicated that children with autism do not acquire language in the normal way, via a gradually expanding system of categories and rules (Roberts, 1989). Instead they learn by echolalia. Chunks of rote learned language are slotted in, with increasing appropriacy, so that, in time, it may be difficult to distinguish between this 'mitigated' echolalia and self-generated language. Those with good cognitive ability may become very skilled at acquiring language in this way, especially when talking about topics which interest them. An example of this facility which caused some amusement to parents occurred during a family trip to the shops. As a traffic warden approached their car, left on a yellow line, their four-year-old daughter, a connoisseur of videos, called out in an impeccable American accent, "Hey, look out, here come the cops!"

It is very usual for children, later diagnosed as having autism, to be seen by a speech and language therapist early on, as language delay is more often than not the cause for initial concern. A developmental approach to assessing communication is essential, and standardized language tests may be relevant. Many parents and carers have unrealistic expectations of what speech and language therapy can offer. Assessment should provide information to enable them to gain better understanding of the nature of their child's difficulties and what may be appropriate in terms of intervention. This may be at odds with their earlier expectations and, indeed, with those of many professionals, for whom one-to-one speech and language therapy is seen as the answer. It is at this point that assessment and diagnosis come together and it is essential that parents are helped to understand the core difficulties of social development which go beyond the acquisition of speech and language. In other words, they need to have the Triad of Social Impairments explained to them, in relation to their particular child's difficulties, and this may be very different from their previous perceptions of autism. (*See page 73 for information on parent workshops.*)

The schedule of the 'autistic continuum' provides a framework for assessing communication that encompasses understanding and expression as well as the *use* of language. Although it is very common for children with autism to show a delay in the acquisition of language, it is not this aspect which is particular to the disorder. Often with more able children, the real problems only emerge after language has developed, when they fail to use it appropriately or for interactive communication. Typically, parents will report that their child has a wide naming vocabulary, although it is evident that it is used inconsistently. There is a pedantic, 'old fashioned' or quaint quality about many of these children's utterances which may be derived from videos or stories, and appeal to them in some way. Although, on standardized assessments of language, able children with autism can score relatively well with age-appropriate comprehension, this does not mean that they will necessarily be capable of understanding in real-life situations. Their understanding tends to be literal and concrete, so that embedded meaning, figures of speech and inference are largely lost on them. An example of this was the response of a very able nine-year-old boy with autism who was offered 'marble cake' as a menu option at school. He became most upset and cried, saying that he could not swallow marbles. Socially normal children would have been able to question this somewhat confusing name for a pudding, and would also have been able to reflect, in the context of their daily experience, that any menu option would be edible.

Some verbal children with autism use their expressive language with great fluency. They are able to talk at length about subjects which are of interest to them, and have a remarkable facility for manipulating any dialogue back to their favourite topic. It is not unusual for young children with autism to show precocious skills in reading and writing, yet it is a mistake to extrapolate from this that such a child is academically gifted. These skills may be islets of ability which do not necessarily develop as expected.

As well as the internationally approved diagnostic criteria for autism, DSM IV (1994) and ICD 10 (1992) which are regularly updated and revised, other classification systems have been developed, such as PL-ADOS (The Pre-Linguistic Autism Diagnostic Observation Schedule) by DiLavore *et al* (1995). In general, diagnostic checklists are useful in identifying autism when it presents in its most classic form. They are less useful in identifying those children whose autism presents in a more subtle way. In addition, there is a distinction between the diagnostic criteria needed for scientific research purposes and the more pragmatic approach to diagnosis based on a child's needs, which is relevant to practitioners such as teachers and speech and language therapists. The experienced practitioner in the field of autism can develop almost a sixth sense or 'gut feeling' about the autistic nature of a child's profile of difficulties, which to others may appear precipitate. Yet this is to misunderstand what assessment is all about. Surely the aim must be to clarify the child's needs rather than to conform to rigid diagnostic criteria which may result in concluding that a child is 'not autistic'. Well, what is he? Does it matter what you call him? What *does* matter is doing right by that child, and ensuring not only that he is understood, but that he and his family have access to appropriate resources that are available in education, health and social services. Because we promote the notion of a *context* of autism, rather than necessarily a diagnostic label, we would encourage professionals to feel comfortable in discussing autism with parents and carers at an early stage, rather than avoiding the issue for fear of repercussions and expensive demands on services.

Checklist

Consider the context of autism if these descriptive traits present in a young child.

▶ Evidence of a lack of interest in other children, so that the child may be described as a 'loner'. Alternatively, he may want to relate to other children, but does not seem to know how to go about it. However, the child may be happy to participate in rough-and-tumble play.

▶ The child does not use language communicatively, despite a good or adequate vocabulary. In addition, there may be snippets of relatively sophisticated language which is derived or learnt.

▶ The child's play is limited, never seems to lead anywhere and has a repetitive quality. The child may also have unusual and/or pervasive interests, which are dominating. There may be an excessive interest in videos, which may be blamed by parents for causing the difficulties.

(*These three areas of difficulty are components of Wing's Triad.*)

▶ The child seems unable to extract meaning from situations and experiences, despite a capacity to acquire knowledge and retain facts.

(*This is evidence of weak central coherence.*)

▶ The child does not display joint attention behaviour, or show awareness of the needs and interests of others.

(*This relates to difficulties with theory of mind.*)

▶ The child is described as 'odd', 'quirky', or 'extremely stubborn' and may be very difficult to manage.

▶ The child may show an extreme attachment to a parent, which may or may not have been preceded by indifference.

CHAPTER 2

Setting the scene for intervention

As we have already pointed out, speech and language therapists are frequently the first professionals to see young children with autism, as it is the failure to develop language which first alerts parents to the possibility that something may be wrong. The expectation is that some treatment sessions will alleviate any problems. They want something done quickly, they do not expect to hear anything seriously untoward and, if they have any doubts, they may have constructed a scenario to explain their child's difficulties, which may sound familiar: "He watched too much television"; "We moved house"; "He reacted badly when his sister was born"; "His father/cousin/brother/uncle didn't speak till he was five." It is not realistic to expect parents to come with an understanding of the relationship between social development and language. The fact that, in addition to language delay, their child ignores other children, has unusual interests, lines up toys and interacts only to obtain his needs is put down to quirks of personality rather than aspects of an underlying problem. To unravel misconceptions and place seemingly disparate strands into a framework puts an enormous responsibility onto the shoulders of the clinician. Any failure to address the underlying nature of the child's difficulties may affect the long-term outcome for the child, and the family's well-being. This may sound alarmist, but nevertheless describes the experiences of many parents who follow false trails and inappropriate remedies because it all went wrong, right at the beginning, when mistaken conclusions were drawn.

Family breakdown is now extremely common in our society, and most children with a less than ideal home background grow up without any particular problems. If there are social or behavioural difficulties, they are not qualitatively akin to autistic spectrum disorders. Yet it is unfortunately not unusual for family problems to be seen as the only possible explanation for the profile of difficulties shown by more able verbal children with autism who come from dysfunctional families. Once family problems become the focus of concern, the child's difficulties are inevitably seen as a corollary to this, and any other possible causes are disregarded.

Since the terminology used to describe children's areas of deficit has changed to accommodate political correctness, it has become far more difficult for parents to understand the implications of their child's problems. For example, the term 'learning difficulties' is used in place of the term 'mental handicap', as are 'learning disability' and 'developmental delay'. Such terms, used for the best possible reasons, can mislead parents by implying that the problems are remediable and will go away. It is important, therefore, to ensure that they are not misled by terminology which can be misconstrued, and that open and honest discussions take place so that parents have a realistic picture of the present situation and the implications for the future.

It is evident, however, that there is considerable inconsistency regarding the issue of terminology since, in a number of journals, particularly those directed towards an American readership (where political correctness originated) terms such as 'mental retardation' and 'mental handicap' continue to be used freely. However, in educational circles, 'learning handicap' and 'developmentally delayed learner' are now favoured.

Making sure that parents have a realistic understanding of their child's difficulties is the first step in the process of intervention. It follows from there that appropriate management of the child's needs, and the family's well-being, are all-important at this stage. Although diagnostic issues may have been clarified, other concerns may need to be addressed, and it is incumbent on the clinician to provide a setting in which parents can do this with confidence. These concerns may range from unsuitable accommodation to genetic counselling, or other medical issues that may have been overlooked, or only recently developed. These might include 'absences', febrile episodes and allergies. No one professional will be in a position to solve all possible problems, but all professionals should be aware of what resources are available and be able to point the family in the right direction.

For example, clinical psychologists have experience of dealing with a wide range of behaviour problems that may be a source of considerable upset within a family. A local Portage scheme, or other home-based intervention programme such as Hanen, if available, may be able to offer support and input to those with a range of more severe difficulties. Parents should be introduced to relevant and up-to-date reading material, so that they are in a position to make informed choices. Libraries and bookshops cannot necessarily be relied upon to stock the most suitable titles. One of the most important and positive actions that can be taken is to ensure that the child has a place in a playgroup or nursery, as it is vital that he experiences social contact with other children. In the United Kingdom it may be appropriate to recommend that parents ask their local education authority to instigate formal assessment procedures which may lead to a Statement of Special Educational Needs. Many authorities now provide an adviser to help parents through the complexities of this process. For some parents, an introduction to a local support group is a life-saver, though for others it is the reverse, since it may confirm their worst fears about the future. This applies just as much to contact with the National Autistic Society, which provides services and information for both parents and professionals.

The lives of some parents and siblings of children with autism can be so fraught and disturbed that access to respite care facilities is a priority. Contact with these services in the United Kingdom may be made through social service departments, or directly in the case of organizations such as Contact-a-Family, Kids or Mencap. Parents should be encouraged to consider these services, if not for themselves, then for siblings who need time and opportunity to engage in activities which are precluded when a brother or sister with autism is around. In some areas, activities and meetings are organized specifically for siblings, and these may be helpful in alleviating the stress and embarrassment often experienced by normal functioning children in the family.

There are parents who, despite all efforts to help them, appear unable to move forward in terms of recognizing and accepting their child's difficulties. They seem to revolve in circles of anguish which lead nowhere. For them, professional counselling may be beneficial, although it may be extremely difficult for them to acknowledge that they are in need of such help.

For a number of historical reasons, speech and language therapists in the United Kingdom have presented a somewhat low-key image of what they have to offer. Caught as they are between health and education, and with limited and even shrinking resources, this is hardly surprising. No wonder that parents are drawn to high-powered intervention programmes, however dubious and/or expensive. A speech and language therapy programme, delivered without razzmatazz and hype, tends to be given little credibility, regardless of the fact that what is being offered is exactly what the child requires — not in terms of 'teaching the child to talk', but in setting the scene for developing communication in the widest sense. We have the skills, but are in the unfortunate position of having little opportunity to foster them. In saying this, we recognize that we are placing demands on a profession which is already wildly overstretched. The implication of this must surely be the need for more specialism, so that resources are put into the development of specific services for young children with autism.

It is evident that there has been considerable improvement in the recognition of autism. However, providing a diagnosis without offering an 'immediate response service' follow-up is seriously inadequate. It is vital that parents are offered not only information but prompt access to services specific to the condition.

Checklist

▶ Have diagnostic issues been dealt with?

▶ Have the parents understood the implications?

▶ Do other referrals need to be made?

▶ Has the child got a place in a nursery/playgroup?

▶ Should the child be referred for formal assessment?

▶ Do the parents have access to reading material?

▶ Are there family issues to deal with?

▶ Would respite care or a support group be helpful?

▶ Is there a need for professional counselling?

CHAPTER

3 Pre-school intervention

Any programme of intervention must take a child's developmental level and particular profile of skills and deficits into account. Those with good cognitive functioning are far more likely to make good progress than those with impairments in this area. With young, newly diagnosed children, it may be difficult to ascertain the extent of a learning disability because of relatively intact areas, especially in physical development, and visual perceptual skills. All young children with autism will benefit from some sort of pre-school placement which may be in a mainstream nursery or playgroup, or alternatively in specialist provision for children with special needs. This will provide an ideal setting in which to observe a child's behaviour and mode of functioning among his peers. Intervention at this stage should take the form of advising the staff on ways in which to manage the child so that he benefits from the experience without unsettling the group and seriously upsetting other children.

Some problems are predictable: for example, apparent aggression in children who want to join in play activity but have no idea how to go about it; mayhem in the home corner, as the child flings everything about, unable to use the equipment appropriately; or an inability to be part of the group because the activities have little meaning, and the child cannot focus his attention on anything other than his own circumscribed interests.

Advice should focus on explaining the child's difficulties in the context of autism, so that the problems are not just seen in terms of naughtiness and acting-out behaviour. This does not of course mean that the problems he causes are any the less intrusive, but they can be tackled in a practical way, for example by securing some extra support for the child. Focused intervention on a one-to-one basis may then be possible, to teach strategies for co-operation with other children, as well as some functional play to enable the child to engage in meaningful rather than destructive activity in the home corner. Children with well developed social skills can sometimes be persuaded to include the child with autism in their games. At key times, when all the children come together for a story or for singing, the child with autism should be encouraged to join the group, if only for a few minutes. Snack time may be a good starting point for this, as food often provides an incentive. Many children with autism need a considerable amount of help to enable them to try new activities and enjoy new experiences. Indeed, resistance to change may be one of the most difficult behaviour patterns to modify.

Children with autism find the world about them confusing. Because they are unable to extract what is meaningful and thereby predict and anticipate events, even the most simple activities are fraught with uncertainty. Many are helped by having a visual prompt in the form of photographs. These can be used singly, or as part of a sequence, to enable the child to gain some understanding of what needs to be done, or what is going to happen next. Family members, pets, shops, homes of friends and relations and family events, as well as the nursery children and staff, can all feature and be used to help a child make sense of his particular world.

In parallel with introducing the child to a social community of other children, much can be done in the home environment by parents and carers. Socially normal young children do not have to be taught to engage with others, they know instinctively how to initiate social interaction which they find rewarding and enjoyable. Even young babies are adept at doing this, and know how to captivate those around them in order to gain a response. This interaction, at a pre-linguistic level, underpins the development of social communication. Because babies with autism do not 'turn on' their parents in this way, the parents, unless they are unusually perceptive, may be unaware of what should be happening and of the incipient problems which lie ahead. By the time their child has a diagosis of autism, they are likely to need help and encouragement to provide the social ambiance in which to develop these very basic social skills. Using lap play with a six-month-old baby is very different from attempting to do this with a four-year-old, yet this may be precisely what is needed if the child is to learn such skills as eye contact, turn taking and focused attention. The actions involved in rhymes such as *Round and Round the Garden, This Little Pig Went to Market, See-saw Margery Daw* and *This is the Way the Ladies Ride* are ideal for engaging a child whose attention span is very limited. Simple board books for very young children can be used to encourage joint attention, focusing and pointing. Looking at books should be developed as a shared activity, not as an opportunity for the child to flip pages and attend to his own agenda — for example, identifying page numbers or particular pictures.

Many useful activities can be developed out of everyday routines, such as bath time, dressing or laying the table. The aim is to encourage and make the child aware of turn taking and reciprocation, at a very basic and practical level. Parents should be helped to understand that this, rather than one-to-one speech and language therapy, is the basis for the development of communication skills. It does no service to parents if professionals promote the idea that they alone have the skills to enable progress to be made. When parents are aware of the pragmatic aspects of communication they are better equipped to feel confidence in the part they should play. It is they who are with their child in natural learning situations and it is these situations, extracting meaning from everyday life, which are difficult for children with autism. Parents may need to be told that this has nothing to do with financial constraints and a lack of resources, but is the most positive way to provide help for their child.

Teaching a child to point is an important way of encouraging communication. Many children with autism will use an adult's hand as a tool to obtain their needs. Clearly, if they learn to indicate these needs through pointing, they will be further along the path towards autonomy. Pointing will enable them to indicate choices and confirm understanding. Although in the early stages it may be necessary to manipulate the child's hand to point, once pointing has been established, there are countless pointing games which young children can enjoy, and many of these are linked with action rhymes and songs, some of which are available in books and on audio tapes.

We have mentioned bath time, dressing and laying the table as possible opportunities to develop early communciation skills. Some parents will need to be shown how they can initiate a simple commentary as they go about these routines, and develop this into a dialogue. Pointing games can introduce a child to turn taking, which, for example in the bath, may be facilitated through splashing and games with bubbles. The bathroom mirror can be used for naming body parts, or for 'peep-oh' games. Items of clothes can be named, and linked to colours. Laying places at the table for the family, as well as visitors, can foster awareness of others and what is going to happen next. The aim of all these activities is to build bridges of understanding for the child about his environment and the larger world about him. Many ideas for simple interactive activities can be gleaned from sources such as books on working with children with disabilities, home-based programmes such as Hanen, Portage (see useful addresses, pages 87–89) and, not least, the clinician's imagination, since books and programmes cannot always be flexible enough to account for the idiosyncracies of an individual child's problems. Even the most skilled and intuitive parents will appreciate having suggestions for intervention in a written form, with scope to enable them to incorporate their own ideas.

Through the work of Simon Baron-Cohen, and the development of CHAT (page 81), clinicians should feel increasingly confident about suggesting a diagnosis of autism as early as age 18 months. However, experience has taught us that to offer a diagnosis without support is unhelpful and potentially damaging. Although this has yet to be proved by research, appropriate early intervention may not only encourage progress in the child, but provide the parents with something that is tangible and constructive. So many parents have expressed their feelings of helplessness when they know what is the matter with their child, but are not offered any practical help and guidance. No wonder they are prey to costly alternative approaches which seem to provide answers.

What a parent requires is a key person with experience of autism, who can answer their questions honestly, put them in touch with other parents if so requested, offer advice on management and education and provide a continuing programme that can be carried out in the child's home and, later, at playgroup or nursery.

Unfortunately, it is very easy for parents of children with autism to misunderstand the intention behind intervention strategies and to believe that, if they are pursued doggedly, their child will catch up and the autism will 'go away'. This is not realistic, and care should be taken that this is not implied, even unintentionally. Intervention will move a child on developmentally and, in addition, should in itself provide parents with rewarding experiences and the confidence to develop skills they did not know they had. Parent workshops may be an effective way to introduce these ideas and explore particular management issues, which may concern problems with sleeping, eating, toilet training and behaviour.

Parent Workshops

Parent workshops may be useful at any stage, from pre-school years to early adulthood. At the outset, regardless of the age of the children, it is really important to encourage parents to join in a 'brainstorming' exercise, the aims of which are to enable them to focus on the nature of their children's difficulties, and their expectations for future progress. (An evaluation form, entitled *How Do You See Your Child?*, and a general information sheet are included in Appendix I.)

Practical arrangements are an essential prerequisite for a successful workshop. It is important to be flexible about the timing in order to maximize numbers attending, as many parents will be working. This means that a workshop may have to take place in the evening or even at a weekend.

The same flexibility needs to be applied to the location. Almost any space will work effectively, provided it can accommodate the numbers attending and has an atmosphere conducive to informal discussion. It could be a private home, a clinic, a school or even a room above a pub. Apart from facilities for making or providing basic refreshments, the only equipment needed is a flip chart, evaluation forms, information sheets, pens and any materials or books that need to be displayed or demonstrated.

Many parents of children with social development problems feel very isolated and value an opportunity to meet others facing the same difficulties. In addition, those parents who are in denial of their child's autism, or those who cling to unrealistic hopes, may be persuaded to review their ideas in the company of others who have more positive and accepting dispositions.

By introducing parents with problems in common, much that is positive can be generated. For example, they may feel motivated to form a continuing support group, they may feel strong enough to lobby for improved facilities for their children, both at the present time and in the future, and they may act as an information network.

●————————————●

The next question is, when is a child ready to benefit from a social skills group? He is not ready if he can only attend with close one-to-one supervision. There must be an ability to focus on activities not of his own choosing. Language comprehension should be at no less than a three-word level on, for example, a Derbyshire assessment (Knowles *et al*, 1980). Pre-school children who satisfy these criteria will be more likely to have developed a level of cognitive understanding which is necessary if they are to benefit from this type of input.

What can be done in circumstances when it is not possible for the child to attend a group for whatever reason? (It may be because of a rural setting with poor transport, no other children with similar difficulties, or even unsuitable premises for group work.) Much can be done in the home by families, if they are supported and shown what to do. While there are some parents who instinctively know how to help their child, others have little confidence and no idea how to begin. The following possibilities should be explored.

1 Ensure that the child has a place in a local nursery or playgroup, which may be receptive to advice on ways in which they can help the child.

2 Is there a local Portage service or other home-based programme which may be relevant?

3 Is there a local toy library?

4 Is there a parent support group either specifically for autism or for more general special needs?

5 Provide parents with titles of books which may be helpful, plus information about the National Autistic Society.

6 Provide parents with ideas for enhancing the skills which underpin social development. They can be expanded and adapted according to the child's changing needs and progress. Advice should always be in writing, and reference can be made to any published material which may be useful to parents.

Introducing a Social Skills Intervention Programme

No intervention programme must be seen or presented as some sort of 'cure' for autism. The aim is to teach the basic strategies for social communication which the child with autism needs help to acquire. These 'learnt' skills need to be practised and developed in real-life situations, at home, in school and so on. This means that parents/carers as well as teachers/therapists have a vital role to play in the success of this type of intervention. However, it is most important to ensure that everyone works to the same agenda — in other words, that parents have realistic expectations of what can be achieved. For those who imagine a rapid advance into interactive conversation, the reality of their child being able to sit still and listen may scarcely rate as progress at all. If it has not been possible for parents to attend a workshop, it is essential that they are offered a session, prior to the start of the group, in order to explain the elements of communication development, and to avoid misunderstandings and disappointment. It is important that they develop some understanding of the underpinnings or 'building blocks' upon which communication skills evolve. The pyramid diagram (Figure 1) could be drawn up on a flip chart to help explain this. It will provide the clinician with a means of explaining why, for example, merely repeating words or having a good memory are not in themselves evidence of the development of communication skills.

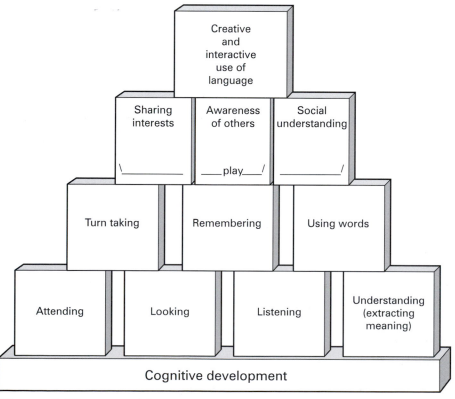

Figure 1 *The pyramid*

A child's cognitive skills will have a direct bearing on the level of social functioning which he can reasonably achieve. In other words, a developmental approach is highly relevant to the teaching of social skills. Not all children with autism will necessarily be suitable candidates for intervention of this kind. If, despite good cognitive abilities, a child's behaviour is consistently challenging or disruptive, to the extent that it affects the successful functioning of the group, it is better to exclude such a child. This should not be seen as a failure on the part of either the child or the teacher/therapist. More success may be achieved at a later date.

There will always be one or two children who have difficulty separating from their parents. It may be quite simple to wean the child away, by allowing the parent to accompany him into the room and to sit close behind the chair where the clinging child should be sitting. As the child becomes interested in the activities of the group, the parent can gently ease him into his own place.

It is always advisable to group children according to their general level of functioning in order to achieve some degree of homogeneity — the right mix. Therefore some sort of evaluation (*see Form 1, page 71*) beforehand is essential, and it may be a good idea to regard the first two or three sessions as a trial period. The size of the groups will of course vary according to developmental stages. In general, pre-school groups should be small, with no more than six children to two adults, plus the rotation of a parent helper, whereas, by later childhood and adolescence, larger numbers will be appropriate in order to facilitate meaningful interaction and discourse in a wider social context. Similarly, there will be variations in the length of time a session will last.

Early Years

We have already stressed the importance of placement in a nursery. In this setting the child should experience some structure so that he is actively encouraged to engage in meaningful activity rather than be left to pursue his own, possibly idiosyncratic and repetitive, interests. The skills gained from attendance at a nursery relate to the aims of a social skills group:

▶ to develop attention control, through good sitting, looking and listening;

▶ to promote awareness of other children in the group, through turn-taking activities;

▶ to focus on the social use of language, through choosing, greeting, requesting and giving;

▶ to build bridges of understanding of the world about them through activities linked to their daily experiences and everyday lives.

Leaving parents and returning to them should be included as an integral part of the sessions. Children need to know where their parents are going to wait, how to say goodbye and greet them, and how to move as a group between the room where they meet and the waiting area, toilet and so on. Moving from one area to another can be controlled by using a rope, with as many knots as there are children: each child walks along holding a knot, and an appropriate song can make the whole thing more fun. Both parents and children need to know how long the sessions will last, and for how many weeks. There must be a goal, not just an open-ended situation. A simple 'time line' (Figure 2) for the children to refer to each week helps to make this meaningful. A 'time line' can be in the form of a long strip of card, marked out in days of the week, with the days that the group meets highlighted in some way. An appropriate picture — a van, a frog, a car and so on — is then moved from one highlighted day to the next, with due ceremony, at the end of each session. The child then has a visual representation of time passing, and can begin to learn to anticipate the future.

Even small children can be helped to organize their own chairs in a circle for the start of a group. To begin with, a chalk line drawn on the floor can focus their attention to where the chairs should be placed, even if it involves physical or verbal 'nudging' to ensure that it is done. Similarly, at the end of the session, chairs and equipment should be put away. These are very useful exercises to enable children to learn to think for themselves and understand how things happen. All too often, professionals do so much to set the scene that children can become passive participants, with little awareness of how they can affect or adapt their environment.

Each of the planned sessions can have a theme, such as home, pets, family or food. Children can be given something to do or find at home between sessions, to make links and foster awareness and continuity. For example, if the theme is bathrooms, they can bring in something to be used there. This will enable parents to play a part in the programme: the 'homework' will provide a framework for them to develop what is being done in the group.

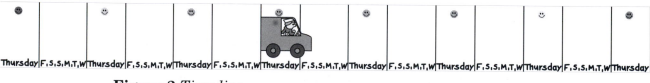

Figure 2 *Time line*

An important component in the organization of the group is the provision of a simple visual timetable, consisting of a series of pictures or photographs that are matched to the sequence of activities within the session. The children are thereby introduced to the idea of 'what happens next?' Difficult behaviour is often associated with a child's inability to recognize this concept. It makes good sense to utilize visual perceptual skills, as this is commonly an area of ability in children with autism. It is up to the professional to decide how to use the picture timetable. In a social skills group, the sequence of pictures will apply to tasks introduced over a relatively short period of time, whereas, in an educational setting, it can be used to show a whole day's programme. Pictograms can illustrate activities such as reading, numbers, language group, computer, play and lunch. Those children who learn to decode print at an early age can be helped to develop understanding by having a written rather than pictorial timetable to refer to. The TEACCH programme, pioneered in North Carolina, has introduced many of these ideas into schools for children with autism in the United Kingdom, with considerable success.

Suggestions for Activities

1 Good Sitting

Start and end each session with up to a minute of listening to soothing music. The children must sit still, hands on laps, and not distract others. This activity provides a trigger for focusing attention. For those children who have real difficulty in sitting still without a high degree of fidgeting, it may be helpful to outline a square on the floor with chalk or masking tape, within which they are asked to keep their feet. At the same time they can be given two soft balls to hold while they sit with hands on their laps. This appears to help such children develop some awareness of what their bodies are doing. Children who find it difficult to remain seated and who jump up whenever they want to say something can be reminded to stay on their chairs by having to support a small cushion behind their backs which will drop down if they get up. These physical reminders can be incorporated into a session as a group activity.

2 Hello Game

The adult says "hello" and names each child in turn, who then has to look at the adult and return the greeting. At a later stage, the game can be developed so that the child who is greeted returns the "hello" and eye contact, then looks at and says "hello" to someone else in the group, who continues in the same way; this goes on until everyone has had a turn. It is important to do this in a random way, so that every child keeps looking, in case he receives the greeting next.

3 Looking at Your Neighbour

A soft ball or bean bag is passed around the group. Each child looks at the person who gives the ball, and says "thank you", before passing it on to the person next to them.

4 Whose Shoe?

Everyone in the group takes off a shoe and puts it in a bag. The bag is then passed around the circle for each person in turn to take out a shoe and decide who it belongs to.

5 Games with Music

These can be musical bumps, statues and hats, follow the leader, with big steps, little steps and so on, or involve copying rhythms and sounds made with simple musical instruments, such as shakers, bells and drums. Action songs and nursery rhymes, especially those with pointing, gesture and simple mime, are useful. Many of these are available on tape commercially.

6 Snack Time

This activity can provide a special focus and an incentive for some children. Serving drinks and small biscuits can facilitate many social skills, such as requesting, responding, saying "please" and "thank you", waiting, turn taking, even clearing up. Each child can have a turn to wear a special apron and be the server. At a later stage choices can be introduced and, later still, children can be given less structure and more choices in deciding for themselves what it is appropriate to take, according to what is on offer. By then group members may be most adept at monitoring each other, and correcting when necessary!

Some children may find it difficult to wait while everyone else is served. Placing all the drinks on a tray once they have been poured discourages grabbing, and makes waiting more meaningful.

7 Cutting and Pasting

The themes of the sessions can be used as a basis for these activities. The children can be helped to work together to produce a simple display or a scrap book.

8 Returning to the Circle

The children are encouraged to run around the room. At the sound of a shaker or drum they have to return quickly to their chairs. Later they can be told to return to a different chair.

9 'You're Looking at Me!'

The adult looks down and hides her eyes. The children in the circle have to look at her. She then looks up and gazes directly at one particular child, who indicates his awareness of this by saying, 'You're looking at me!' or simply 'Me!'

10 Where's the Sticker?

A child is taken out of the room and has a sticker put somewhere on his clothes or body that is clearly visible. When he comes back, the other children have to say where the sticker is.

11 Turn Taking Exercise (1)

Find a toy which is popular, such as a little man who can be placed at the top of a ladder, to wobble down. Each child has a turn to use it, just once, and then allow the next child to have a turn.

12 Turn Taking Exercise (2)

Place a selection of farm animals in a box. To the accompaniment of *Old MacDonald Had a Farm*, each child has a turn to take out an animal, which is then used in the next verse.

13 Turn Taking Exercise (3)

Ring a Ring a Roses, with one big chair, and enough small chairs for the rest of the group. Instead of 'falling down', everyone sits down on a chair. The question is then asked, "Who's sitting in the big chair?" Everyone then has to point and say the child's name.

14 Turn Taking Exercise (4)

Turn taking can be made more meaningful for some children by the introduction of a simplified version of the 'Mexican Wave'. Children in a circle raise and lower their hands in a sequence, one after the other. As one child's hands go down, the next one's hands go up.

15 Cooking

In one of the later sessions, 'Snack Time' can be linked to a simple cooking activity, so that children can appreciate the connection between making something and then eating it. Melted chocolate mixed with rice crispies is all that is required. Choosing fillings and making little sandwiches is another possibility. It is always advisable to check with parents, in advance of these activities, whether a child is allergic to any foods.

16 Looking at Books

As mentioned earlier, there are any number of delightful, well illustrated books available for young children. Books with flaps to look under may be especially useful, since they can incorporate turn taking.

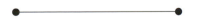

These are but a small selection of possible ideas, given in no particular order, that can be used with groups of young children with autism. Many more can be invented or adapted and the possibilities are endless. Bear in mind that mayhem may ensue because, for instance, a child or children refuse to have their shoes taken off, or react adversely to particular sounds — the possibilities for subversion are also endless!

It goes without saying that free play is an essential element of any group work with young children and time should be allotted to some free play activity. Children can be helped to get the idea of shared play activities: they can be asked, "What do you want to play with?" and "Who do you want to play with?"

Some children may need a lot of help in this area to develop what can be best described as 'functional play'. Although they may do very well in the structured group activities, they are at a loss when left to their own devices, and have little idea how to make use of play equipment. Some children, overwhelmed by the lack of structure and the presence of their peers, may become disruptive and overexcited. Once they have been helped to use toys more purposefully, there may be much progress. Play routines using dolls, dressing-up clothes, tea sets, cots, kitchen utensils and so on can be taught to enable children to occupy themselves more meaningfully. Although this will not lead to the development of creative and imaginative play, it is possible for children with autism to extend their play repertoire, to some extent, and to gain pleasure and enjoyment from doing so. Parents benefit too, from seeing their child involved in normal play activity, even if it is somewhat repetitive.

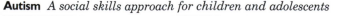

Checklist

▶ Are there children requiring a social skills group?

▶ What are their cognitive levels?

▶ Do any have severe behaviour problems?

▶ List those with broadly similar needs as possible candidates.

▶ How long should the group last (length of sessions, number of weeks)?

▶ Have the aims of the group been clarified to parents?

▶ List possible activities under headings, such as looking, listening, turn taking.

▶ Plan specific themes for sessions; link them to 'homework'.

▶ Make a time line and visual timetable.

▶ Organize snack time, avoid additives and be aware of possible allergies.

▶ Send out relevant forms *(see Appendix I)*.

Statementing

As the child approaches statutory school age (in the United Kingdom), it is essential to ascertain whether formal assessment procedures have been instigated, with a view to obtaining a Statement of Special Educational Needs. There is considerable variation in the speed and efficiency of local educational authorities (LEAs) and the ways in which they act. Although it is required that the process be completed within a prescribed period, there is ample opportunity for stalling or delaying the start of the process, so that many parents suffer seemingly unending stress and frustration in their attempts to gain recognition of their child's difficulties.

Clinicians who have worked with children in social skills groups will be in a strong position to provide information which will be relevant to this process. Firstly, they can use this information to nudge the authority into action when nothing appears to be happening. Secondly, they will be in a good position to offer constructive advice about the kind of school placement that will benefit the child. However, this may require considerable tact if parents are to make the right choices. Some parents are reluctant to acknowledge that their child has special needs, and they will express a conviction that, once the child is in a mainstream school, any difficulties will disappear. Perhaps these parents need to have it pointed out that, in the present climate of financial constraints, the LEA will be only too happy to defer spending money supporting their child, but this may not be in his long-term interests. It is a fact that, unless there is some specificity in the wording of reports prior to statementing, the LEA will be unlikely to respond positively. Use of such phrases as 'difficulties with social communication' are much too vague and may be applied to children with a wide range of problems. Realistically, it is far more likely that the child will get the help he needs if there is a reference to the presence of autism.

Other parents, while acknowledging their child's difficulties, are unwilling to consider anything other than a mainstream placement and feel that, with full-time support, this will ensure the best outcome. They will use arguments about learning from other children, good role models, being accepted and so on. But is this really so? Unfortunately, in the 1980s, Special Education in the United Kingdom suffered an image crisis, when expertise and good practice were set aside in the quest for integration, a move understandably taken up with enthusiasm by parents with these views. (The publication in the United Kingdom of the green paper *Excellence for all Children*, October 1997, has once again raised integration issues.) Attendance at a special school was regarded as a stigma, which would set a child apart from society, and many LEAs closed down their special schools for political as well as financial reasons. At first the provision of classroom support for children with Statements of

Special Educational Needs in mainstream schools was reasonably generous. However, demand escalated and now there is a reluctance to meet these burgeoning costs, resulting in a need to reduce the number of statemented children and offering less support to those with statements.

Integration is far more complex than many parents care to admit. Children with autism cannot absorb social competence simply by the proximity of socially normal children, and they can be more isolated and stigmatized in a mainstream school than in an undervalued special school, where they stand a better chance of being fully assimilated into the school community. All too often, their difficulties prevent them from being accepted by other children, and they may become victims of teasing and bullying. It should also be borne in mind that, in the real world, teachers in mainstream schools with large classes will have considerable difficulties in modifying and adapting the curriculum, the classroom and the playground to suit the needs of children with autism. Parents should be encouraged to consider their children's long-term happiness above everything else. Even academic achievement may be a heavy price to pay for sacrificing this. However, it is possible to compromise, and this will be considered from different perspectives in Chapters 4 and 6.

There is of course another scenario, where parents want their child to have a special school placement but nothing suitable is available within the LEA. It is beyond the scope of this book to discuss the protracted battles that can ensue between parents who demand placement in a special facility elsewhere and an authority which is determined not to spend the money. There are no easy answers to any of these issues, and compromise on both sides may be the only solution. Some of the agencies which can assist parents in their quest for an appropriate educational placement are included in the list of useful addresses in Appendix II.

4 Infant-level intervention

At this stage (age 4/5 to 7 years) children with autism will have started school. They may be in a mainstream setting with or without support, depending on whether the school has agreed to put the child forward for formal assessment, which may or may not lead to a Statement of Special Educational Needs. Parents must expect this process to take some time, since a code of practice with specific stages has to be followed. However, some schools are prepared to act quickly if they are aware of a diagnosis of autism. Alternatively, children may be in a special school or unit. The setting will have some bearing on the type of intervention that is possible.

In a special school setting it is easier to organize groups, as social skills training can be timetabled as an integral part of the school curriculum, and may well feature as a component of a child's Individual Education Plan (IEP). In this setting, the groups can be ongoing, and more flexible, with the added advantage that this sort of provision is not seen as something clinical that goes on elsewhere, with little reference to education. Teachers and classroom assistants can be valuable partners in the groups and ensure that there is a carry-over from the structured social activities to more general classroom and playground behaviour. They will also be able to provide feedback on individual children's progress or particular difficulties. The obvious disadvantage of groups in special schools is the familiarity factor: children will know each other too well, and there will be little incentive to develop and explore wider social contacts.

It is much more difficult to set up groups for individual children attending different mainstream schools. The timetables in the schools may make it extremely difficult to bring a number of children together at a time which suits everybody, and it may be impractical to consider after school time for younger children, who are not at their best at the end of the day. A suitable mix of children is more difficult to arrange, and travel and transport problems may be insurmountable for some families. In addition, many clinical premises are either unsuitable in terms of size or are not 'user-friendly' for a variety of other reasons.

However, there are ways to circumvent many of these problems. For example, it may be easier to include some mainstream children in an established group within a special school or unit. All the participating children benefit from this and it makes the group less 'clannish', enabling the special school children to accommodate newcomers and widen their social experience. As well as being comparatively easy to facilitate, because the groups are already in existence, this sort of arrangement promotes closer liaison between different types of schools, and can be regarded as an example of good 'outreach' practice. Bear in mind, however, that the mainstream newcomers will require extra attention at first while they adapt and catch up with the others, who may have established skills which they have yet to acquire.

When the social skills groups are clinic-based, it is essential that contact be made and maintained, not just with the children's parents, but with their teachers. (A contact letter and pamphlet are included in Appendix I.) The work of the group should be linked to the child's daily life, both at home and in school. Without making these connections, the group is in danger of becoming an end in itself, with no clear objectives. There must be indentifiable short-term goals that can be achieved during the period that it runs. If the child has learnt the meaning of good sitting, looking, listening and turn taking by the end of the group, then a period for the consolidation of these skills is necessary, with the possibility of another group some time in the future, to move the child further on.

This all sounds extremely time-consuming. However, the aims of the group can be circulated in written form at the outset and a follow-up report and advice sheet provided for both school and parents when the group ends. Any adult who is actively involved with the child should be invited to attend one of the sessions to appreciate what they can do to reinforce what is being taught.

At infant level, it should be possible to initiate a somewhat more structured approach to the teaching of social skills. Since there is no point in reinventing the wheel, the introduction of Wendy Rinaldi's excellent 'Social Use of Language Programme' (SULP) for primary and pre-school children (1994) has much to recommend it, whatever the setting and, to date, it has not been bettered. The programme features friendly monsters who display both good and bad social skills in simple illustrated stories. Children with autism, who are often particularly interested in monsters, readily identify with such characters as 'Betty Butting In' and 'Tommy and Timmy Taking Turns', among others, and really enjoy listening to and talking about their predicaments. The programme has already been extended to deal with topics relevant to older children, such as bullying in the playground and making compromises. As well as reinforcing the basics of good communication skills, the programme enables children to recognize their own shortcomings, by association with the actions and behaviour of the characters in an engaging way. Once children have learnt what 'good sitting' and so on mean, it is possible to use the phrase, 'I want to see good sitting' as a trigger or code for achieving the required behaviour. This approach is more constructive than negative criticism, which may well be meaningless to the child. Positive behaviour is promoted through posters which illustrate the skills being aimed at and the awarding of chart stickers at the end of sessions enables the participants to reflect on their own achievements. Assessment charts are included with the programme, so it is possible to monitor children's individual progress. However, the photocopiable assessment chart (Form 5 in Appendix I) is more specific to autism and may therefore be more useful.

The programme provides a framework around which other activities can be introduced. It does not have to be followed slavishly — indeed, it is important to allow for a degree of spontaneity, because this is more akin to what happens in real life, and because it makes the sessions more interesting for everyone! The pace of the sessions and the type of activities introduced can reflect children's individual needs and interests.

A particular aspect of language which often causes problems is the understanding and use of question words. A developmental approach with much repetition and practice can really make a difference. In general, 'What?' is easily understood, and the majority of able children with autism will have a good naming vocabulary, produced in response to 'What's this?' Therefore 'Who?' is a good starting point, and any number of games can be devised to encourage children to link the word with particular group members. 'Where?' usually produces the automatic response of 'there!', and it may be some time before children get the idea of being more specific, and explaining, 'under the tree', 'on his lap', 'behind the chair' and so on. The intention must be to enable the child to appreciate that other people may not know what he knows. It is a good idea to send one child out of the room and then get another to explain on his return where a hidden object can be found. Such games may reveal that some children find prepositions confusing. They are often helped by the use of simple manual signs, such as Paget-Gorman or Makaton, which are visually clear and explicit. Once children become aware of time, the use of 'When?' can be explored. Initially, it should be linked to familiar events such as birthdays, and culminate in thinking about the past and the future. 'Which?' can be explored on the basis of making choices. It may be necessary to leave 'Why?' and 'How?' until a later stage, if the child's understanding remains limited.

The following session plan for about an hour and a quarter has been used with groups of able five- to seven-year-olds, and may serve as a model for up to eight children, with two adults.

Suggested Session Plan: Infant Level

1 Children arrive and arrange chairs in a circle.

2 'Good Sitting': children are required to sit still and listen to music for a few minutes.

3 'Hello Game': ensure that everyone has a turn and check eye contact.

4 'News Time': keep it simple; everyone has to say something. If necessary, use a home/school diary or information given by parents to make this possible *(see page 49)*.

5 SULP story: start with 'Looking Luke', with a discussion at the end. Children are given posters to take home and colour.

6 Work on 'Theme of the Week'. This could be a sensory project, such as tasting, which would involve sampling different foods and developing the appropriate vocabulary such as sweet, sour, crunchy, spicy and so on. Another topic could be feeling: children will enjoy using a 'feely bag' to develop appropriate vocabulary, such as rough, smooth, soft, hard and so on.

7 End this part of the session with a repeat of 2.

8 Children are asked to reflect on what they think they did well. Give out stickers, to be put on a wall chart.

9 'Snack Time'. Children are chosen in turn to be the 'Server' and wear a special apron. They are helped to sort out the number of cups, types of drinks and snacks, and request jugs of water. The others are expected to arrange the table and chairs. Ensure that the children observe rules of social behaviour, say 'please' and 'thank you', and wait for everybody to be served.

Snack time is most valuable and fulfils a number of different purposes. Firstly, it is very popular and, coming at the end of a session, provides an incentive for good behaviour. Secondly, rotating the role of 'Server' emphasizes turn taking in a meaningful way. Additionally, the use of eye contact, the making of choices and the acquisition of socially appropriate language are all reinforced. Not least, it encourages awareness of the needs of others, which is fundamental to social understanding.

10 At the end of the session, children clear away and replace chairs and tables.

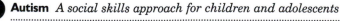

More Ideas for Session Themes

▶ Textures

▶ Concepts of size

▶ Concepts of position

▶ Clothes — what do we wear and when?

▶ Animals and pets

▶ Our families

▶ Rooms in the house

▶ Gender and pronouns

▶ Food

▶ The weather

▶ Birthdays and festivals

Speech and language therapists who are organizing mainstream groups in the community for only a limited time, ideally eight weeks, may want to break down the suggested plan in more detail. Nevertheless, this must not be done at the expense of flexibility and spontaneity. It is also important that the children's parents are kept fully informed about the aims of the group, the skills that are being introduced and the general format of individual sessions. Samples of a detailed session plan (Form 8) and a handout for parents (Form 9) are included in Appendix I.

Common Problems

Aggression

Attempts to bring about changes in behaviour should always be linked to the circumstances and situations in which the behaviour occurs. We have already suggested that telling a child with autism that he is naughty is unhelpful. Not only is it unlikely that he will really understand the concept, but the disapproval inherent in the use of the term is likely to have a negative effect and foster poor self-esteem. It is far more constructive to help a child understand what led up to his outburst, and why his behaviour was unacceptable. For example, a child who had been excluded from a mainstream school was invited to join a class in a special school for a few minutes, as he had arrived early for his social skills session. Although he sat down, apparently happily, he soon became disruptive and had to be taken out when he scratched the classroom assistant. When his behaviour was discussed with him, it was suggested that, if he had not liked being in the class, he could have asked to go back to the speech and language therapy room. He therefore had to learn to recognize his own feelings before he could learn strategies to deal with such situations in a more appropriate way. Children with autism find it very difficult to reflect on their own behaviour and, for this reason, they may respond well to rules presented in a direct and straightforward way, without wordy explanations.

Having said this, they also have to be taught that rules do not apply for ever, and there has to be some flexibility according to circumstances. For example, a child who has been taught to wash his hands whenever he uses the toilet also has to learn, when out for a picnic, not to make a fuss because there are no washing facilities behind the bushes.

Some children with autism show marked changes in their behaviour from one month, week, day, or even hour, to another. Despite attempts to link the changes to particular events or circumstances in the child's life — even allergic reactions — nothing emerges to make sense of them. The only explanation appears to be fluctuations of mood ranging from a seemingly depressive state to one of being 'hyped-up' and manic. While in these extreme states, the children may be all but impossible to manage in any kind of group and require one-to-one attention. This contrasts with their comparatively amenable and co-operative behaviour at other times.

Anxieties

Children with autism are especially prone to anxiety, which is not really surprising since they lack the ability to extract meaning from situations and to ask appropriate questions for reassurance. It is very difficult indeed to disentangle the origins of extreme anxiety which may occur in seemingly innocuous circumstances. It is not unknown for the anxieties themselves to become the focus for intervention, which tends to happen when the child is seen by a professional with little experience of autism. This can have a disastrous effect on the family, if it is implied that the causes are linked to poor parenting and unsuccessful management, rather than a developmental disorder with biological origins. It is not acceptable to explain the triad of social impairments in terms of emotional conflict or even deprivation. This may have the effect of delaying action on appropriate educational placement and denying access to a range of support services and resources.

Repetitive and Ritualistic Behaviour

This type of behaviour, common among children with autism, has been explained in a variety of ways, but perhaps makes best sense when considered within a framework of weak central coherence and sensory deficits. These disabilities lead to impairments of awareness and understanding; the child with autism will have difficulty in predicting outcomes and events, which results in anxiety and insecurity. It is not surprising that repetitive stress-reducing behaviours are adopted as coping strategies for situations that are not understood. Once such patterns of behaviour are established, they are extremely difficult to eradicate.

Postscript on Emotional and Behavioural Problems

Children with autism can have emotional and behavioural problems, in addition to their social impairments. They are as subject to family break-up, abuse and unhappiness as any other children. However, approaches for addressing these problems which may be appropriate for socially normal children are unlikely to be so for those with autism. In addition, it is important that professionals are not so diverted by family problems that the co-existence of autism goes unrecognized.

Checklist

▶ Consider suitable candidates for a group.

▶ Where are you planning to hold it?

▶ Can any of the candidates be integrated into an existing special school group?

▶ Who will run the group with you? Options: in school, teacher/classroom assistant; in clinic, SLT/assistant/student.

▶ With mainstream children, have you liaised with Special Educational Needs Co-ordinators (SENCOs)*?

▶ Has a meeting been arranged for parents, to explain aims?

▶ Consider asking parents to sign a contract. (*See Chapter 7.*)

▶ Plan the content for eight sessions/one school term, including a choice of themes.

▶ Assess children using a record chart.

▶ Plan follow-up procedures, including evaluation forms. (*See Appendix I.*)

▶ Do any children display emotional/behavioural problems, anxieties or aggression? Do they require special referrals?

* In the UK, all mainstream schools have a designated teacher whose role is to support children with special needs. These are referred to as SENCOs.

CHAPTER

5 Junior-level intervention

At this stage (age 7–11 years), the aim will be to consolidate and reinforce all the groundwork that has been introduced at infant level. However, there will be children who have missed out on social skills input earlier on: perhaps they have only just been diagnosed, or have recently transferred from a mainstream school to a special school. Clearly, they will need to be taught the underpinnings of social communication which have already been described before they can proceed further. One way of dealing with this situation is to appreciate that it does no harm for the experienced members of the group to revise what they are supposed to have learnt. The pace of the revision will be faster than the first time round, and will provide an opportunity to review levels of progress in individual children. It is unlikely that boredom will be a problem; after all, this is an area which is particularly difficult for them, and much practice is needed in a variety of situations. Frequent reminders about good sitting, looking, listening and turn taking will always be necessary, and these skills must be established, before it is realistic to move on to more subtle aspects of social functioning.

The expectation is that, having acquired some ability to monitor their own conduct, albeit in a functional way, they are now being encouraged to consider other people's needs, and to start to see how their own social behaviour can impinge on others. At this level, their appreciation of others' needs is also at a functional level; for example, they know that other children have different preferences in relation to drinks, snacks and television programmes, but will have very little, if any, understanding of other people's states of mind. A practical way to approach this is to develop *the concept of manners*. Children will already know about saying 'please' and 'thank you', but the concept means much more than this. Manners represent the way we get on with other people and involve a range of social behaviours including conduct, courtesy and demeanour, not simply politeness. It is possible to present these rather abstract ideas in simple terms which are relevant to daily life experiences of the children in the group, and this should be done in stages.

Stages for Introducing the Concept of Manners

Stage 1

Discuss bad manners with the group and invite them to share their ideas. They will get a lot of fun listing antisocial behaviour such as burping, farting, coughing and sneezing over other people, picking noses, and so on. From this jokey beginning, children are encouraged to think about how they feel when they experience others doing these things at close quarters. This may well be something that they have never considered before, and the discussion can be focused on the notion of the 'yuk' factor, and things that are 'rude'.

Stage 2

Move on to discuss good manners and compile a list, which will probably include general politeness and terms such as 'sorry' and 'excuse me'.

Stage 3

Develop the idea that manners do not matter if you are all by yourself. From here the link is made between manners and getting on with other people.

Stage 4

At this stage it is worth making use of children's books on the subject of manners. A number are available (see 'Useful Books and Equipment for Intervention' in Appendix II). They provide a very useful introduction to the subject and encourage children to begin to think about others: for example, not waking a baby, tidying up, not talking in the cinema, and so on. Discussion helps the children to focus on reasons why things like this matter: a woken baby may cry, tidying up is a way of helping and talking in the cinema means that other people cannot hear properly. These are things that are not difficult for children to understand and relate to their own lives.

Stage 5

By now the children should be ready to appreciate at least some of the content of the excellent books by Aliki. One, entitled *Manners*, is particularly useful at this stage. It expands on the ideas included at Stage 4, and contains a wealth of materials to enable any teacher or therapist to explore a wide range of issues concerning social behaviour as well as moving them on to think about feelings. Role-play and modelling can be introduced as enjoyable ways in which to make the concepts meaningful.

Stage 6

The subject of feelings is an extremely important aspect of social understanding. Children will readily identify happy and sad, but the range of feelings that they should be taught to appreciate must be considerably wider than this. A game to introduce the idea of showing and identifying feelings can be played by getting children to recite the alphabet, or a nursery rhyme, in voices that suggest anger, fear, tiredness or boredom, excitement and so on. Two other titles by Aliki, *Feelings* and *Communication*, will be useful at this stage and can also provide a framework for role-play.

Progress has to be made through making links with real-life experiences. Information provided by the child, or by parents, should always be utilized to illustrate particular feelings. For example, feeling 'disappointed' can be identified with the cancellation of something the child was looking forward to; 'scared', with something frightening that was seen on television; and 'excited' with anticipation of a birthday or holiday. From learning to identify their own feelings, children can move on to think about how other people may be feeling.

Children with autism are never going to be intuitively perceptive about their own or other people's feelings. However, it is possible for them to acquire some understanding through cognitive processes and this may enable them to pursue happier and more fulfilled lives.

Body Language

Children can learn to identify feelings by observing body language. At first it will be necessary for adults to model this for the group. At a later stage, when children have grasped the idea that different parts of the body can indicate how someone is feeling, they can be encouraged to demonstrate this for themselves. This can be done, using a sheet, to show, in turn, just faces, hands or feet. Facial expressions are the easiest for others to recognize; gestures and movements with the hands or feet alone are more subtle and may need some thinking about. For example, thumbs up, waving, wringing or drooping hands give very different messages and, similarly, dancing, kicking and stamping feet also convey information about feelings.

Dealing with Particular Problems

Information from parents can also be extremely useful for working on particular problems or behaviours which are a cause of concern. For example, a parent reported great anxiety about her daughter's fascination with fire. This information provided the stimulus for group work on thinking about and discussing 'dangerous things'. This proved to be a very effective way of dealing with this problem.

Individuals with autism can be helped to modify their behaviour by the introduction of social stories as suggested by Carol Gray in *The New Social Story Book* (see 'Useful Books and Equipment for Intervention'). The stories should include descriptive, perspective and directive elements, athough it is important that there is only one directive element in each story. Here is an example.

> I like to play with my friend.
>
> My friend likes to play with me.
>
> We have fun together.
>
> If I hurt my friend, she will not play with me.
>
> I will play with my friend and be kind.

Visual Strategies for Improving Communication by Linda Hodgdon (see 'Useful Books and Equipment for Intervention'), provides a wealth of ideas for dealing with children's individual problems. For example, the universally known symbol of a red circle with a line through it can be used effectively to communicate 'no' in many different situations.

Suggestions for Role-play

Children with autism are known for their ability to memorize, and role-play provides them with 'scripts' to enable them to cope with situations that are likely to recur. Adults leading the group can model both good and bad behaviour or manners, which children can discuss before trying things out for themselves.

Examples for Scripts

1 The child is offered food he does not want or like.

2 When not to comment on a person's appearance.

3 How to apologize.

4 How to ask to borrow something, or to ask for something back.

5 How to say 'thank you' when you don't like what you have been given.

6 What to do or say if you are bullied.

This list can easily be extended and can include ideas from both school and home.

Work on manners and feelings can easily provide material to fill an eight-week social skills programme for those working in a clinical setting, as well as those in a more flexible situation within a special school. There should be continuous consolidation of all the basic work introduced at an earlier stage. For example, there is no point in repeating the 'Hello Game', when the group have become really slick in passing on their greetings in this sort of way. At this stage, it is important to adapt the game to reflect the progress that has been made, and to introduce a range of greetings to accommodate real-life situations. When they come into the room, children should be encouraged and reminded to greet those present. Initially, this may be simply "Hello", with eye contact. Older children can be encouraged to use a wider range of appropriate expressions, such as "Sorry I'm late", "Happy New Year", "Did you have a good holiday?" or "Are you feeling better?" At the end of the group session, other appropriate expressions can be practised: "See you next week", "Have a nice holiday" and so on.

News Time

'News Time', which was introduced at a simple level for infants, can now be developed and expanded for junior age children, to enhance their awareness of the world about them. In addition, it encourages them to think about other people's experiences and to recognize that this may be of interest to them. Adults in the group should also have a turn to tell news, especially as they are in a position to provide a model for the way it should be done.

There are many inherent benefits to be gained from 'News Time'. It encourages turn taking and listening skills (children should be asked to recall the subjects of the rest of the group's news) and alerts them to current events that they may have heard about on television. This is a very natural way to stimulate simple discussions, and encourages children to ask each other questions. This may be the time to introduce 'Why?' and 'How?' (see Chapter 4). Because children with autism tend not to show curiosity, they are often ill-informed about matters that are relevant and important to them. In the absence of their enquiries, adults frequently overlook the necessity to brief them about things that are going to happen, such as temporary staff changes in school, illness and absences, and so on.

'News Time' is a practical way to address the problems of mentalizing and lack of coherence which are fundamental in children with autism. They begin to appreciate that, unless they explain something that has happened to them, nobody else in the group will know anything about it. In addition, they begin to become aware of the relative importance of their individual topics of news, and to realize that certain items are of more significance than others. Reporting that they had smoked salmon sandwiches for lunch, in the week that they moved house, or acquired a new baby brother, may typify this problem. Parents therefore have an essential role to play by providing information about their child's experiences so that he can be cued in to those topics that are the most important. However, it is vital to let the child know how this information was obtained: for example, "Your mum told me that you went to the cinema last week!" If this is not done, the child will not develop an awareness and understanding of what other people may or may not know.

Initially, a lot of help may be needed to enable children to understand that talking about the same topic every week, even if it is of great interest and importance to them, may be boring to others. Similarly, they have to know when they have said enough. A useful way of helping children to judge when they have talked too long is to slowly unwind a ball of string while each member of the group has their say. The relative lengths of string can then be compared and the owners of very lengthy, or very short, pieces can be encouraged either to contract or to expand their output!

Contrary to the traditional view of the remote autistic child who avoids all physical contact, in reality, many will flop over other people, touch, poke, hug or even pinch, unless prevented from doing so. This behaviour can be very disturbing and disrupting in a group, especially when the child being assailed is one who is really upset by such intrusions. Not only is it extremely important to inhibit this behaviour because of its disruptive effect, but it is essential to set boundaries while the child is of a manageable size, since such behaviour in older children and adults is not only inappropriate, but can be construed as threatening and open to misinterpretation.

Young children can be taught to appreciate the idea of *own space*. It can be explained that everybody needs a space around them and no one else should come inside it unless that child wants them to or asks them to. It is easy to illustrate this: the children are encouraged to identify their 'own space' by extending their arms in front of them with finger tips touching, and then moving their arms backwards in a circular movement, so that elbows rest close to their bodies at waist level and hands pointing forwards about 15cm from their sides. The concept of 'own space' presented as a rule is more meaningful and positive than repeatedly reminding a child to leave someone else alone. As children get used to the idea of own space, they can be taught to be more flexible. The circle they draw with their arms can be reduced to reflect the fact that sometimes they have to sit closer together. But the rule still applies!

'Own space' is an important concept to take beyond the group. This particularly applies to the playground, where many children with autism have difficulties, either because they invade other children's space or because they have no strategies to deal with the intrusion of other children, whose intentions may be far from benign. In the latter case, children can be taught to seek help. However, they also need to learn to recognize friendly approaches, and not to overreact if they are accidently pushed by another child.

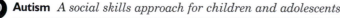

Sequencing and Memory Games

The following are useful for filling in when there are some odd minutes to spare.

▶ *Kim's game.* A selection of objects on a tray are displayed for a short time and then covered over. The children are asked to recall the objects.

▶ My granny went to market and bought . . . . / In school I might use . . . . / I went on holiday and took . . . .

▶ An object is passed around the group, and each child adds some information about it in addition to what has already been said. The information must be relevant and refer to colour, shape, texture, smell, composition, use and so on.

Story Sequences

Story sequences, using picture cards, can be a very useful activity for children from about junior age onwards. However, it would be a mistake to assume that, because a child can order a series of picture cards, he necessarily understands the essence of the situation that has been illustrated, as he may be reliant on superior observational skills. It is as well to encourage the child to make a comment about the overall situation depicted, for example, 'A little boy is lost', 'The family is at the seaside' or 'It's about a birthday party', before he is asked to sort the pictures into a story. This means that the child is encouraged to extract meaning and make sense of the whole, rather than focus on details which may not be relevant to the story. This exercise links to the inherent difficulties with central coherence experienced by individuals with autism (Frith, 1989, Happe, 1994). There are many attractively produced resources available for this kind of activity. (See Winslow, LDA, Appendix II.)

Showing Photos

Children in the group can be encouraged to bring in photographs which they would like to show other people. They might choose pictures of themselves as babies or young children, family groups, events, pets or holidays. The photographs can be used to elaborate on the people and events shown. The aim is to enhance the group's understanding of time and relationships, as well as situations and occasions, which may not be part of individual children's experiences.

Issues for Group Management

At the outset, it is necessary to discuss with the children why they are coming to the group. It is not unknown for some of them to refer to their own autism as a reason, but they may be unable to explain what this means. To develop their understanding, a good starting point could be to talk about what they as individuals have in common. This can be explained in simple terms, such as "You find it difficult to know how to behave with other people", "You find it difficult to know what other people mean or are thinking", or "You don't find it very easy to make friends."

In conjunction with this, it is important to acknowledge children's developing maturity by keeping them informed of changes in the group, which may concern new staff, new children coming and others leaving. This has the effect of making them feel part of a group, and aware of their own and others' individuality. Once again, the right mix of children in terms of cognitive functioning and behaviour is vitally important. One disruptive child who is unable to modify his behaviour will influence other vulnerable children, and undermine a successful outcome for the entire group. What can be done about this problem?

First, decide whether the child is really unable to participate, or is simply unwilling. If it is considered to be the former, there is no point in trying to make him fit into a situation that he cannot cope with, and it is far more constructive to recognize that he is not ready for this approach. It can be tried again at another time, and meanwhile it will be more helpful if other strategies are explored — for example, those used with younger children.

Second, the unwilling child needs a different approach. His behaviour may be a learnt response to any new situation, and obviously this possibility will need to be checked with those who are familiar with him. Attending the group should be presented as something special, and he should be made aware that certain standards of behaviour are implicit if he is to share the 'treats' aspect. It is to be hoped that the child will get enough of the flavour of the group session to enable him to want to be present and not cause problems for other children. If he does disrupt the group, exclusion must be the sanction used. Repeated warnings quickly lose any impact and, in effect, disrupt the harmony of the group. It is far preferable to explain calmly to the child that you feel very sorry, but he is spoiling the group for others and will have to leave because of his behaviour, and that you hope this will not happen again next time. It is for such situations that another adult is vital — so that the child can be removed to an alternative location and provided with a mundane activity which is not highly rated for interest and enjoyment. The child should be welcomed back on the following occasion and, if his behaviour is satisfactory, should be praised in a

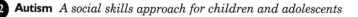

positive way, not in terms of an improvement on what happened before, but by saying how pleased everyone is to have him back in the group again. This strategy has proved to be effective with many able but disruptive children. (See Chapter 6 for behaviour management in general.)

Third, it is not unusual for a particular activity, for example action songs, to trigger disruptive behaviour in an individual child who is otherwise manageable. The reasons for this may not be clear, but the situation needs to be dealt with promptly, in order to limit its effect on other children. Stopping the trigger activity and moving on to something different is often the simplest solution and highlights the importance of flexibility in group management. Even the best planned programmes may need to be modified, and it is important that the group leader has the ability to respond spontaneously to situations as they arise.

Checklist

▶ Are all the children in the group at about the same level in the development of social skills?

▶ Have the basic skills of good sitting, looking, listening and so on been established?

▶ Is the group ready to move on to the concept of manners?

▶ Plan a programme of intervention to include role-play.

▶ Are Aliki books appropriate?

▶ How can 'News Time' be developed? Do children prioritize their news, talk too long, talk only about their own interests, and so on?

▶ Is the group ready to discuss the reasons for their attendance?

▶ Is the group briefed on changes and events, and encouraged to ask questions?

▶ Is there a policy for managing the group and dealing with disruptive children?

▶ Liaison with parents: are they kept involved by being provided with information about their child's particular problems and progress?

6 Intervention with older children & adolescents

Structured schemes such as Wendy Rinaldi's *Social Use of Language Programme* (NFER–Nelson, 1992) are relevant and useful at this stage. Within the framework of assessment and short- and long-term goals, children are encouraged to consider and practise interactive aspects of communication, linked to particular situations such as introductions, giving directions, enquiring about others' feelings, taking messages and asserting rights. However, as children mature, it will be increasingly important to extend social skills training into the realm of *life skills*. The individual strengths and weaknesses of group members should be used to provide an ethos of shared support, so that particular problems and experiences that may occur outside the group can be included to reflect what actually happens in real life: for example, problems with bullying, other people's expectations, and anxieties about particular social situations.

While the NFER SULP programme is particularly useful in providing a framework for working with older children with autism, it is by no means the only source of ideas; some other sources are listed under 'Useful Books and Equipment for Intervention'. As we have already mentioned, the important thing to bear in mind with any programme is to take out of it what is useful and relevant and not feel that it has to be followed slavishly to be of any value. Indeed, very productive sessions can develop spontaneously out of particular circumstances: the consideration of actual experiences is always going to be more meaningful than any contrived situations. Time must always be made to talk about changes, upsets, quarrels and bereavements, as well as positive things, such as success and achievement — all the substance and reality of people's lives. It is invaluable to give young people with autism the opportunity to think about things which they would not normally consider or even know about. In a sense, the aim is to teach them some aspects of theory of mind and, although it would be over ambitious to believe that this could be a panacea to solve all their social difficulties, it can be shown to make a real difference and can enable them to cope with life more successfully.

Always bear in mind, when working with children with autism, that it is important to give mental states meaning and substance. Information must be made explicit in the context of learning; never assume that things have been understood, or even that the children will be able to tell you what it is they do not understand. Often their speech is associative, and the surface messages should not necessarily be taken literally. This compounds the difficulties involved in trying to sort out problems when they arise. Understanding people with autism has been likened to understanding individuals from a very different culture. We should be aware of the great efforts they have to make to understand us and to adapt to our expectations.

Idioms, Inference, Metaphor and Jokes

We must emphasize, however, that it will only be those with good cognitive skills who benefit from this approach, whereby an intellectual process is substituted for a skill that is largely instinctive in socially normal people. Even the most able individuals with autism may find everyday idiomatic expressions perplexing because they have connotations linked to class, education, fashion, age and so on, the subtleties of which are beyond their comprehension. The introduction of idioms should be tackled from the aspect of understanding, rather than use, as there will be many pitfalls in attempting to introduce them appropriately into social conversation. How do we know when phrases in common use become passé? When did 'smashing' lose out to 'wicked'? When did 'mutton dressed up as lamb' metamorphose into 'past her sell-by date'? The understanding of social conversation can certainly be enhanced when idioms and metaphorical figures of speech are recognized as important elements of communication, although embedded in seemingly throw-away remarks of other people. The following list of examples may be helpful:

▶ bend over backwards,

▶ the last straw,

▶ draw a blank,

▶ catch red-handed,

▶ get the hang of it,

▶ down in the dumps,

▶ cut and dried,

▶ raining cats and dogs.

Another aspect of social communication which can be tackled in the group with a lot of fun is jokes. There are a number of suitable books available, and for older children it is possible to discuss what jokes mean — again, so that they are understood rather than as something that should be memorized and repeated at a later date. If children can be taught to recognize when a joke is a joke, social interaction is going to be a lot less fraught for them. Nevertheless, however much is taught, inference and implied meaning are always going to be difficult for people with autism, but it is worthwhile to provide them with some props, rather than none at all.

News Time

It is worth continuing to develop 'News Time', and the ranking of news according to its relative importance. Children should be made aware of the distinctions between personal news and school news, in contrast to news that is of national or international importance. Awareness of the range of news items that may be discussed can encourage young people with autism to think beyond their own particular preoccupations. It is possible for them to develop some awareness of what may be boring to others, and to learn to recognize at least some of the signals displayed when a listener has lost interest.

Sometimes particular news events, rescues, robberies, even murders, which children have seen on television will catch their attention. These can be used as topics for general discussion, to develop their understanding of real situations, especially when they are upsetting and worrying.

Appropriate Behaviour

This issue is a complex one, increasing in importance as children reach adolescence, and perhaps expect to enjoy more freedom and independence, and to take part in youth culture. It encompasses their own behaviour and also the behaviour of others towards them which aims to ensure not only their psychological well-being, but also their physical safety. Their needs reflect socially normal young people, but they require considerably more explanations and guidance to help them to make the transition from childhood. Earlier work on the concept of manners can now be broadened considerably to enable them to make the changes.

It is to be hoped that they have already been encouraged to shed behaviours which, as they get older, could be embarrassing or misconstrued, such as touching and hugging people indiscriminately. While eccentric behaviour can be tolerated or even indulged in young children, it may appear altogether different, if not threatening, in a large adolescent. We cannot emphasize enough the importance of eradicating, as much as possible, behaviours which could lead to problems. These may not be major issues — indeed, parents may be inured and hardly notice them — nevertheless, they mark the child as 'different'. Such habits as licking hands, smelling people, fiddling in trousers and so on should all be firmly discouraged.

Concerted effort by school and home is usually successful in inhibiting these inappropriate behaviours, especially in more able children. However, they may recur at times of stress and anxiety.

Role-play

By this stage, children who have taken part in social skills groups at an earlier age will have become familiar with the idea of role-play, in terms of memorizing useful 'scripts' for particular circumstances. This can now be developed to cover more subtle and complex situations. Children without previous experience may find it difficult to cope with this without some sort of induction into what is expected of them. For example, simple mime guessing games can be extended into dialogue and working with another person.

Because the majority of children are avid television viewers, they do not generally have much difficulty getting the idea of pretending to be someone else. However, the point of the activity is to get them to develop their 'performance' into the expression of something personal to them. As they become more experienced in this skill, it may be possible to introduce an interpretive aspect so that children become aware of the possibility of there being more than one way of handling a situation. This may not resolve their difficulties, but should lessen some of the inevitable confusion in their lives, and at best give them strategies for coping.

Ideas for Role-play

1 *Negotiation in the family*   This is very useful to start with, as the lives of many adolescent young people with autism are organized totally by parents and there is little opportunity for autonomy. A simple example may be that a young person wants to try a different hairstyle. How can this be brought about? The number of family issues that can be tackled are manifold!

2 *Negotiation in the community*   This can include asking for things that are not on show in the supermarket or ordering food in outlets such as MacDonalds, including what to say if given the wrong order. More ideas of this kind can be found in the NFER SULP programme.

3 *White lies and excuses*   People with autism tend not to be capable of telling lies; indeed, their honesty is a common source of their social difficulties, as they have no natural compunction to refrain from telling the naked truth. Hence the range of anecdotes reported by parents of both embarrassing and droll comments made by their autistic offspring. A teacher at the end of a particularly hard day did not feel any better after being told by a pupil, "You're looking pasty, my dear." Little scenarios can be developed on the lines of the scripts referred to in Chapter 5.

4 *Showing sympathy and concern*   It would of course be unreasonable to expect young people with autism to show these feelings naturally in a socially appropriate way. In fact, the reverse may be the case. For example, concern about someone's problem, illness or loss may result in repeated questioning which only exacerbates a situation, despite the fact that the intentions were entirely laudable. Perhaps discussing the loss of a pet can be the starting point for learning how to express sympathy, and thinking about the upsets and sensitivities of others. People with autism may have the capacity to show sympathy, even if they cannot empathize. Scenarios could include comforting a 'friend' who is crying or inviting a newcomer to join a group activity.

5 *Assertiveness*   Role-play is an ideal way to practise such skills as giving and receiving compliments, standing up for oneself, making suggestions, disagreeing and complaining, asking for clarification and apologizing. If the young people gain confidence, it may be helpful to use a video recorder, so that group members can evaluate their own 'performances' and learn how to make changes.

●━━━━━━━━━━━━━●

If children cannot cope with role-play activities, it is possible to convert these into turn-taking games. For example, giving and receiving compliments, as mentioned above, can be organized at a simple observational level. Everyone sits around in a circle, and has a turn saying something nice about another child's appearance, clothes, skills and so on.

Growing Up: Learning to Make Choices

This aspect of group work is very much linked to the acquisition of life skills, and is usually included in the school curriculum. In the United Kingdom, it is in the National Curriculum as part of personal and social education. It can provide many enjoyable activities, while teaching useful ways and means of being more grown-up and participating in teenage culture.

Parents of children with autism often have mixed feelings as their offspring move towards adulthood. It is one thing to accept a child with disabilities, but quite another to acknowledge an adult with disabilities. Indeed, it may reopen forgotten feelings of disappointment and even anguish. For such reasons, there is sometimes an unconscious desire to prolong childhood, and not encourage a son or daughter to present in a way which acknowledges their developing maturity. This may be seen most clearly in choices of clothing. Obviously, it is important not to offend parents if a 'Thomas the Tank Engine' T-shirt is to be put aside by a 14-year-old, in favour of a more age-appropriate logo. If parents are happy to co-operate, going to the shops, as well as choosing items from a catalogue, can be extremely helpful. The underlying aim is to teach appropriateness.

Another aspect of this can be exercises on selection of presents for family, friends and, perhaps, other members of the group. These activities can be presented as an outing to local shops, or in a variety of games and projects, including the following.

1 Using mail order catalogues, cut out pictures of clothes or presents suitable for different categories of people, such as grandparents, mothers, fathers, peers or babies. A more advanced stage would be the selection of items for people in the group, taking personal preferences into account.

2 Using pictures again, pretend you are going away for a week. What things should be packed?

3 Selecting clothes for particular situations and weather.

4 Which shop or shops would you go to to buy clothes for yourself? Or to buy books, toiletries, games, and so on?

5 Visit the local chemist and choose three things girls or boys might use, or be interested in using, such as deodorants, shaving kit, shampoo, aftershave or perfume. Which things would you choose for yourself?

6 Select an appropriate place to have a drink, an ice cream, a burger, a curry, and so on.

7 Locate the police station, bus stops, station, post office and public telephones, and so on.

8 Practise using public telephones and taking and leaving messages.

9 Work out routes, and how to get to places.

10 'Favourite Things': discuss, for example, football teams, food, countries to visit, bands, videos or television programmes. (This activity can be adapted to suit younger children.)

11 'What Would You Do?': a good starting point would be to look at a situation and consider a number of different ways of dealing with it. Situations can be presented through magazine pictures, episodes from television 'soaps' and real life. Commercially produced material is available from educational suppliers. (See 'Useful Books and Equipment for Intervention', in Appendix II.)

All these activities will encourage young people to be more aware of their surroundings and to move towards greater independence.

It may be worth considering linking up with a local secondary school to develop a joint social skills programme. Not only is it likely that they will have children with autism in the school, but they may also have children with other special needs who would benefit. Many SENCOs welcome opportunities to participate in ventures of this kind and, for special school children, a weekly visit to a mainstream school will be a stimulating experience. Similarly, vulnerable mainstream children may enjoy spending time in a smaller and more personal special school environment.

With greater independence comes the question of personal safety, which has particular relevance to socially naive people, who may have difficulty assessing the character and motives of others. Inevitably, if and when they are out and about by themselves, whether they are male or female, they will be vulnerable. It is beyond our brief to explore this important matter, but children do need to have strategies for dealing with untoward situations. Role-play may again be very useful, in teaching how to say 'no' and reporting worrying incidents to known and trusted adults.

Social difficulties inherent in autism will not go away, but can be improved by working developmentally and systematically through issues as they occur. It is through working in a group that young people learn to cope with the quirks, vanities and insensitivities of others. Young people with autism need to be made aware that some adults they come across may be mean and horrible, and behave badly. This should be linked to understanding that sometimes, when things go wrong, it may be the adult who is at fault.

Checklist

▶ Consider the cognitive levels of the group when planning sessions.

▶ Are any of the published social skills programmes (SULP, for example) relevant to the group?

▶ Are there any particular problems among group members which can be worked on?

▶ Consider any inappropriate behaviour among group members which should be tackled.

▶ Consider how role-play can be used effectively in the group.

▶ Move on to life skills — what aspects can usefully be addressed? Liaise with parents and school staff.

▶ Discuss the imperfections of society in general: rudeness, unkindness and intolerance of others.

▶ Consider planning a social skills programme for an academic year. For example:

Term 1 Work on feelings, identifying states of mind, body language and so on.

Term 2 Work on 'what words mean'. Consider idioms, metaphor, jokes and so on.

Term 3 Practical life skills exercises in the community.

7 Further practicalities of running social skills groups

When a group is up and running, there has to be a measure of spontaneity in making use of situations as they arise. It is, however, essential to spend time beforehand in planning and preparation, especially when working with children who are not in special education. It is reasonable to assume that, within special schools, social skills training will be part of the general curriculum, and no particular arrangements will be necessary.

Location

Have suitable premises been located in which to run the group? The size of the room needs to be considered, as well as furniture and facilities for both the children and their parents or carers. Bear in mind that a clinic waiting room will not be suitable for working with a group of parents. Easy access via public transport must also be an important consideration. It is worth thinking beyond a community clinic or health centre, to other venues such as nurseries, schools or family centres.

Paperwork

If a rolling programme of social skills groups for pre-school or mainstream children is envisaged, it is essential to have a reliable referral system, which will identify those who are likely to benefit from this type of input. A model referral form (Form 1), which sets levels of functioning as a prerequisite for inclusion in a group, is included in Appendix I. The criteria can be adapted and modified to suit particular circumstances.

Once the logistics of the group have been arranged, and suitable children identified as possible candidates, it will be necessary to contact parents or carers. This is not simply in terms of offering an appointment or block of treatment, but rather as a contract which involves them making a commitment. Realistically, unless parents can make a commitment, this kind of intervention is not viable. At the outset, the onus is on the organizers to make this clear so that, if a place is accepted, parents will be obliged to play an active part, by attending the parents' sessions and ensuring that their child attends the group every week (see Appendix I for a suggested letter format

(Form 2), which includes an agreement about making video recordings of group sessions).

In order to evaluate the effectiveness of a group, it is essential to have a rapid means of assessment to provide a baseline, and for monitoring progress. This can be used at the initial and final sessions, as well as for long-term follow-up. In addition, it can serve as a record sheet for each child, so that continuing observations can be documented while the group is running (Form 5). This form is presented in an extremely simple way, as the pressures inherent in running groups often make detailed record keeping impractical. As an alternative, however, weekly session plans can be copied and then used to record individual children's responses to particular activities.

Forms can be issued for parents to complete, describing their own perceptions of their child's difficulties and their expectations of the group (Form 4). At the final session, they can re-evaluate these perceptions and comment on any changes (for better or worse) which they have observed in their child (Form 6). Some parents may prefer to complete this form anonymously, for whatever reason. In addition there is a form for use by professionals who may wish to comment on any observable changes or progress in children they are working with (Form 7). All these forms which are included in Appendix I should provide a framework for audit and information in terms of collecting data for measuring outcome. In general, the forms are not suitable for secondary-aged children.

Use of Video

A certain amount of thought needs to be given to the purpose of using video recording. With young children, it can provide a very useful means of monitoring progress. Video can be used to demonstrate ways in which to facilitate appropriate behaviour. Absent parents can see what went on in the group, and share in their child's participation. In addition, video provides a professional with a useful training tool for demonstrating the value of social skills groups.

Older children can be encouraged to assess their own performance through the use of video and, indeed, may become quite adept at using camcorders themselves. They may enjoy acting out little scenarios for role-play and even make judgements about their own shortcomings, if not those of their peers!

Camcorders can also be used to make simple 'films' about topics that are being explored by a group, or are of particular interest. For example, a film could be made about preparations for a particular event, about an outing, or a school journey, or even about home life, or pets — in fact any topic which lends itself to recall, reflection and discussion.

Human Resources

In Chapter 3 we referred to the ratio of adults to children in the running of groups, and how this will vary according to the ages and needs of the particular children. The type and frequency of any input for parents must also be considered in terms of the number of professionals needed. Students and assistants can certainly play a part in the running of groups, but should not be put in the position of having to support and advise parents.

Although a social skills programme is essentially directive and structured, the individuals leading the group must not only be able to hold the children's attention, but have almost a sixth sense in recognizing when things are not working. They must be capable of switching to different activities to suit the tenor of a particular session. Often, the children respond best to leaders with good performance skills, who are able to 'act out' meaning and feeling in an explicit way. It is helpful if the adults running the group can decide in advance which of them will present particular activities. This enables the children to have a better idea of who to direct their attention to. It also makes good sense because it enables the non-active leader to concentrate on observing and recording any relevant information about individual children's responses.

When introducing parents as helpers or observers to the group, care must be taken to set clear guidelines for their involvement. Some will find it very difficult not to interrupt, either to reprimand or to encourage their own child. Therefore it is important to advise them that for the duration of the session they should relinquish their parental role and allow those running the group to manage their child. It is also to be expected that some children will become more difficult when their parent is present.

It may be advisable not to include parents in groups for older children, not least because the promotion of independence will be central to the ethos of the group. Some parents may find it difficult to accept this, seeing it as a form of exclusion. It may be helpful to explain to them that normal social development includes activities in which parents have no part. Parents of children with disabilities often find it difficult to stand back from their children. Having protected and possibly fought for their needs over many years, they fall into the habit of organizing their children's lives to a degree which 'normal' young people would not tolerate. It is of course appropriate to keep parents informed of what goes on in the group, especially as they will have to help their child with 'homework' tasks. Copies of session plans can be used to put parents in the picture. They will need to know, not simply the range of activities, but their purpose: for example, that snack time is not just a refreshment period, but an opportunity to practise turn taking, making choices, requesting, using appropriate behaviour and language, considering the needs of others and interacting with peers.

Duration of a Group

It should be borne in mind that, even with pre-school children, each session should last for at least an hour. If parents have been asked to make a special commitment to bring their child to the group, they should also get something out of it for themselves. A good hour, with a cup of tea, in the company of other parents with similar problems, can in itself be beneficial. A varied selection of activities, supplemented by snack time, will almost certainly require between an hour and an hour and a half. It is not difficult to vary the pace, on days when sluggishness and non-co-operation prevail, with play, both indoors and outdoors, listening to music or even blowing bubbles.

Final words

We are not researchers and are not involved in projects to determine the nature of autism; nor are we in a position to explore theories which explain the variability of the condition. However, our extensive practical experience does enable us to examine the research of others and to assess its relevance.

In particular, the research into central coherence and theory of mind, while not explaining everything about autism, has enhanced our understanding of the disorder. Indeed, it has enabled us to gain new perspectives and develop ideas for programmes of intervention which address the intrinsic problems.

Because, in the past, children with autism were described simply as 'autistic', there was an assumption of uniformity. Even current literature reinforces a stereotypic picture. Yet, in reality, children with autism differ from each other, in the same way as socially normal people do. Their personalities, their families, their educational and life experiences will all make for differences, so that, despite the common thread, each one is a unique individual. Progress, and eventual outcome, will be influenced by these factors, as well as those more directly linked to the diagnosis of autism.

In recent years, a number of very able people with autism have written and talked about their difficulties from the inside, and it is apparent that their progress and achievements are hard won. These achievements have nothing in common with the succession of 'miracle cures' for autism which continue to be publicized in the media. Despite the very real advances in understanding the nature of autism, the mythology persists and, at regular intervals, programmes and news items appear describing autistic children who have been cured in an amazing variety of ways, from dog ownership to swimming with dolphins.

We would like to re-emphasize that the ideas and approaches described in this sourcebook do not constitute any sort of 'cure' for the condition of autism. We would claim, however, that it is possible to effect real changes and improvements in those children who have autism and good cognitive skills, for the simple reason that they have the capacity to learn at least some of the social skills which most people absorb with little effort, or even awareness. We are indebted to the adults who have shared their experiences so openly with us, and to the children who have participated in our groups and given us so much enjoyment alongside the hard work.

APPENDIX I
Forms & handouts

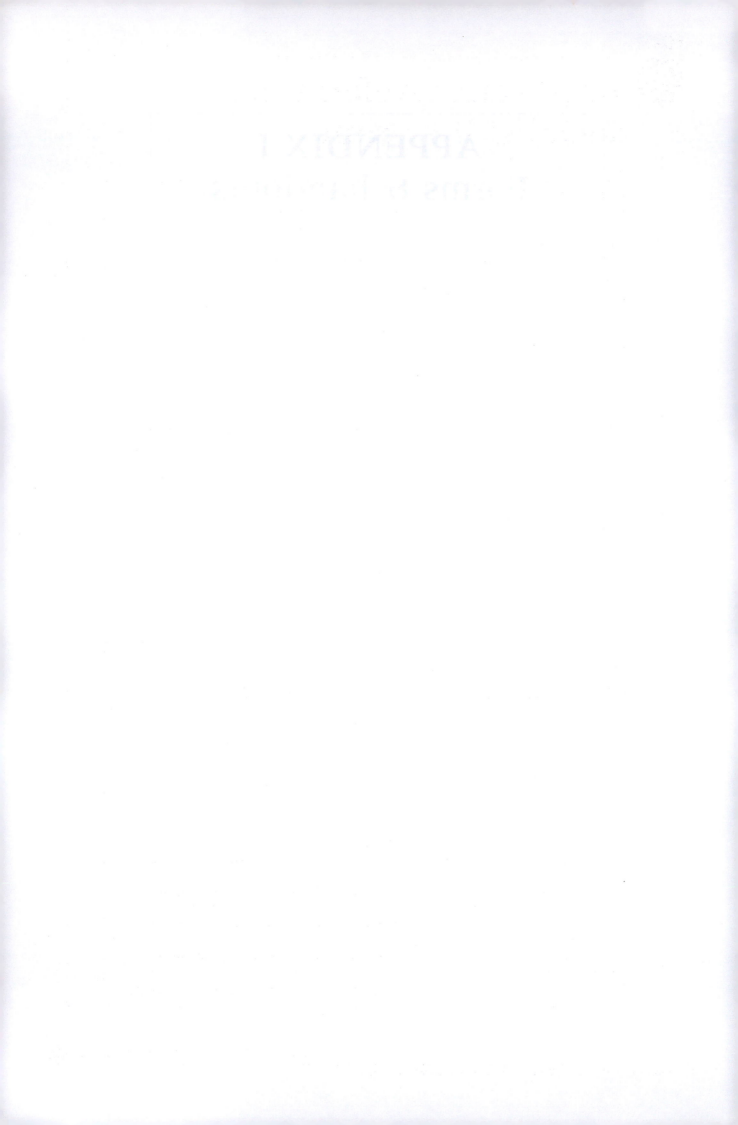

Application/referral for social skills group

Referred by *eg. SLT, HV, Cl. Psych., Ed. Psych. (please denote)* **Date**	
Child's name	
DoB	
Address	
Post code **Tel. no.**	
School/Nursery/Playgroup *NB Child must be in school/nursery/playgroup, and be able to separate from parents.*	
Family doctor	
Priority rating	
Outline previous SLT input	

Other relevant information *eg. medical history, travel difficulties*

Attention level *(please tick)*	**Level 1** ☐ **Level 2** ☐ **Level 3** ☐ **Level 4** ☐
Language level *(please tick)*	**Level 1** ☐ **Single word comprehension**
	Level 2 ☐ **2 – 3 word comprehension**
	Level 3 ☐ **3 – 4 word comprehension**
	Level 4 ☐ **Higher-level language difficulties**

Letter to parents

Date: _____

Dear _____

We are pleased to offer your child _____ a place in a Social Skills Group at the above location. The group will meet for _____ sessions on _____ from _____ to _____ starting on _____ and ending on _____.

As places in the group are limited and we have a waiting list, it is essential that parents only accept a place if they feel able to commit themselves to bringing their child to all sessions. Occasionally a child may not settle in a group, or may find it difficult to cope if he/she is not yet ready for this type of input. In such circumstances, we may suggest that the child is withdrawn.

There will be a Parent Workshop Session to discuss the aims of the group at _____ on _____ from _____ to _____.

It is essential that you attend this session.

Please sign and return the slip below by _____.

We do hope your child will be able to attend.

Yours sincerely _____

. . . .

To Speech & Language Therapy Service

_____

_____

Re: Social Skills Group — dates: _____ to _____

I would/would not like my child _____ to attend this group,

and I will/will not attend the workshop session.

I understand that video recordings may be made of some of the group sessions.

Signed _____

Name of parent _____

Contact telephone no _____

Parent workshop social skills group

Information

The aim of the group is to develop your child's social understanding and use of language.

Many of the children attending the group will have a good naming vocabulary, and may be able to use quite advanced language when making comments, or talking about things that are of interest to them. However, their language has a learnt or derived quality, and may include snippets of videos and echoed phrases which they find pleasing in some way. It is the conversational and interactive aspects of communication that present problems for them.

In order to develop social communication skills, group activities will focus on listening, appropriate looking and eye contact, attention fixing and turn taking. 'Snack time', when a drink and biscuit will be offered, will be an important component of the sessions. It encourages children to make choices and develops their awareness of the needs and interests of others.

If your child has any food allergies please let us know.

You will be invited to participate in a group session, if appropriate, to observe the activities so that you can reinforce them at home. You will also be asked to co-operate in simple 'homework' tasks/course work, and to talk about the group with your child in between sessions. After the last group session, you will have an opportunity to discuss your child's progress, and a brief written report will follow.

We hope there will be liaison with your child's school/nursery/playgroup,* as social skills and social communication need to be encouraged and developed at all times, and in all situations.

The workshop is an opportunity for you to share your concerns about your child, which will help us to address his/her particular needs.

* Delete as appropriate

Parent workshop

How do you see your child?

Date _____

Name of child _____

Date of birth _____

School/nursery _____

1 What do you feel is your child's biggest problem in relation to communication?

_____

_____

2 What other difficulties give you cause for concern?

_____

_____

3 Is it difficult to manage your child's behaviour?
(Please describe.)

_____

_____

4 What would you like your child to gain from attending a group?

_____

_____

5 What do you hope to gain for yourself?

_____

_____

5 Progress profile

Rating scale: 1 = Poor attention/lack of co-operation
2 = Variable attention/co-operation
3 = Sustained attention/co-operation

Child's name _____

Willingness to participate:

Date:		Date:		Date:		Date:	
Scale:		Scale:		Scale:		Scale:	

Date:		Date:		Date:		Date:	
Scale:		Scale:		Scale:		Scale:	

Attention control:

Date:		Date:		Date:		Date:	
Scale:		Scale:		Scale:		Scale:	

Date:		Date:		Date:		Date:	
Scale:		Scale:		Scale:		Scale:	

Turn taking:

Date:		Date:		Date:		Date:	
Scale:		Scale:		Scale:		Scale:	

Date:		Date:		Date:		Date:	
Scale:		Scale:		Scale:		Scale:	

Response to/interest in other children:

Date:		Date:		Date:		Date:	
Scale:		Scale:		Scale:		Scale:	

Date:		Date:		Date:		Date:	
Scale:		Scale:		Scale:		Scale:	

Overall behaviour:

Date:		Date:		Date:		Date:	
Scale:		Scale:		Scale:		Scale:	

Date:		Date:		Date:		Date:	
Scale:		Scale:		Scale:		Scale:	

Comments

_____

_____

_____

_____

_____

Summary of progress

_____

_____

_____

_____

_____

Recommendations

_____

_____

_____

_____

_____

Social skills groups: Evaluation form (parents)

Name (optional) _____

1 Did your child enjoy the group? _____

2 Does he/she ever talk about it? _____

3 Does he/she ever refer to the aims of the group (good sitting, looking, listening, turn taking)? _____

4 Do you feel that the group was helpful? _____

5 Did you find the Workshop session helpful? _____

6 Did you gain anything from meeting other parents? _____

7 Has anyone mentioned progress made by your child (eg. class teacher, grandparents)? _____

8 Have you any comments or suggestions to make? Our service is always keen to respond to parents' views. _____

_____

_____

_____

9 If a further group was offered, would you like your child to attend? _____

10 On a scale of 1–10 (10 = excellent) how would you rate the value of the group to:

You? _____

Your child? _____

Thank you for taking time to complete this form. Please hand it in to the Speech & Language Therapist or, if you prefer, send it to:

_____

_____

_____

⑦ Social skills groups: Evaluation form (professionals)

Name of child _____

The above-named child has recently attended a _____ week social skills group.

In order to monitor his/her progress, it will be helpful if you could complete this questionnaire. The parents know that we are contacting you.

1 Were you aware that this child was attending a social skills/speech and language therapy group?

_____

2 Have you noticed any changes in this child over the past few weeks in relation to:

(a) Communication?

_____

(b) Play?

_____

(c) Relationships with other children?

_____

(d) Motivation and task completion?

_____

(e) Ability to attend and focus?

_____

3 Any comments:

_____

_____

Thank you for your help. Please return this questionnaire in the SAE which is enclosed.

Session I *Observation/self-awareness/awareness of others*

1 Introductions: why are we here?	*Giving information/listening*
2 Make name badges (use for game at end of session).	*Reinforcing*
3 Establishing group rules:	*Thinking of others*
(a) Good sitting. (b) Good looking. (c) Good listening. (d) No interrupting. (e) How to ask for help.	
4 Make a poster for display. Everyone writes their name, or draws their face, with help. Incorporate above rules.	*Co-operative activity*
5 What does our group look like? (a) Recall our names. (b) Say one thing about our neighbour.	*Self-awareness and observation*
6 SULP story: 'Looking Luke'.	*Listening/reflecting*
7 Looking/observation games: Making changes.(Child changes appearance, others identify change.)	*Turn taking*
8 Snack time. Choice: orange/blackcurrant, biscuit. Set rules for this part of the session.	*Turn taking, making choices*
9 Calendar; recall of names.	*Planning and memory*
10 Homework: each child draws a picture of himself, or brings in a photo the next week.	

Handout for parents

Session I *Observation/self-awareness/awareness of others*

ACTIVITIES	SKILLS
1 Introductions	*Giving information*
2 Making name badges	
3 Establishing group rules	*Thinking of others*
4 Making a poster	*Interaction*
5 What does our group look like?	*Recall and observation*
6 Social Use of Language Programme (SULP) story about looking	*Listening/reflecting*
7 Looking games	*Turn taking*
8 Snack time	*Requesting information*
9 Calendar; recall of names	*Planning and recall*
10 Homework: please encourage your child to draw a picture of himself/herself or find a photo, to bring in next week	

We would like to thank Dr Simon Baron-Cohen of the University of Cambridge for allowing us to include the CHAT in this book.

The CHAT
(Medical Research Council Project)

To be used by doctors or health visitors during the 18 month developmental check-up.

Child's name: _____ Date of birth: _____ Age: _____
Child's address: _____
Telephone number: _____

Section A; ask parent:

1 Does your child enjoy being swung, bounced on your knee, etc?   YES   NO

2 Does your child take an interest in other children?   YES   NO

3 Does your child like climbing on things, such as up stairs?   YES   NO

4 Does your child enjoy playing peek-a-boo/hide and seek?   YES   NO

5 Does your child ever PRETEND, for example, to make a cup   YES   NO
of tea using a toy cup and teapot, or pretend other things?

6 Does your child ever use his/her index finger to point, to   YES   NO
ASK for something?

7 Does your child ever use his/her index finger to point, to   YES   NO
indicate INTEREST in something?

8 Can your child play properly with small toys without just mouthing,   YES   NO
fiddling or dropping them (eg. cars or bricks)?

9 Does your child ever bring objects over to you (parent), to   YES   NO
SHOW you something?

Section B; Doctor or health visitor observation:

i During the appointment, has the child made eye contact with you?   YES   NO

ii Get child's attention, then point across the room at an interesting
object and say, "Oh look! There's a [name a toy]!" Watch child's face.
Does the child look across to see what you are pointing at?   YES   NO[*]

iii Get the child's attention, then give the child a miniature toy cup
and teapot and say, "Can you make a cup of tea?" Does the child
pretend to pour out tea, drink it, etc?   YES   NO[**]

iv Say to the child, "Where's the light?" or "Show me the light."
Does the child POINT with his/her index finger at the light?   YES   NO[***]

v Can the child build a tower of bricks? (If so, how many?)   YES   NO
(Number of bricks: _____)

[*] (To record YES on this item, ensure the child has not simply looked at your hand, but has actually looked at the object you are pointing at.)

[**] (If you can elicit an example of pretending in some other game, score a YES on this item).

[***] (Repeat this with "Where's the teddy?" or some other unreachable object, if the child does not understand the word 'light'. To record YES on this item, the child must have looked up at your face around the time of pointing).

Social skills groups: Letter/SENCO

Date: _____

To SENCO _____

School _____

Name of child _____

This child has a place in a Social Skills Group at _____

for _____ weekly sessions lasting about one and a half hours. These will

start on _____.

The group will focus on aspects of social communication such as:

- Self-awareness and awareness of others
- Listening
- Turn taking
- Observation and looking
- Group interaction skills

We hope that you will be able to support _____

in using these skills in school.

You will receive information sheets either directly, or via the child's parents. A
report will be written after the last session, and you will be asked to fill in a
form to enable us to ascertain whether progress has been made. From then on
we will liaise with you, to consider any future needs the child may have in
relation to social skills.

Speech and Language Therapist

Social skills groups: Handout *How teachers can help*

1 While the child is attending the group it might be possible to encourage him/her to talk to you a little about the weekly sessions. We can provide you with information about their format, as can the child's parents. You can simply remind the child of his/her attendance at the group by mentioning the therapist's name.

2 Encourage the child to report back to the group about something he/she has succeeded at in school. Say: "You can talk about that when you give your news." The child's parents could be involved with this in order to make it work.

3 Children with social communication difficulties often find it easier to elaborate on someone else's statement than answer an open-ended question, eg. "I expect you have been to your group this week ... did you play any good games?" rather than "What did you do at your group?"

4 If possible, reinforce the concepts of 'good looking' and 'good listening' at appropriate times in the school day. The child may be helped if he/she is reminded at the start of an activity such as assembly, circle time, news time, story time and so on.

5 Using the child's name before making a request or suggestion helps to focus his/her attention on what is required.

6 The use of phrases such as 'good looking' and 'good listening' is specifically applied in order to try and promote positive reinforcements for acceptable behaviour.

7 Children with social communication problems often have fluctuating attention, and so find it easier to respond to simple rule-based approaches that do not involve convoluted explanations.

8 The child may not see the point of pleasing the teacher, and so needs clear and simple explanations of what is expected in terms of his/her behaviour.

9 Often the child will find the unstructured situations in school, such as playtime, difficult to cope with, especially if he/she finds social interaction difficult. Suggestions as to what games could be played, which areas of the playground have special designations, who to go to for help and so on, might help to diffuse problems. Similarly, the child might need to have the format of 'wet play' made clear.

10 Children with social communication difficulties often have a poorly developed idea of 'what happens next' and the sequence of the daily timetable. They may be helped if they are prepared for changes in advance with very simple explanations that emphasize 'before' and 'after' and are linked to their specific roles, eg: "After you have finished you will be able to …"

11 Changes in the school day, visits, outings, end of term parties and so on, may also need to be presented to the child in advance with very simple explanations. Changes in routine are often treated with suspicion by children with social communication difficulties.

12 Some children with autistic spectrum difficulties have well developed specific skills, eg. computers, reading, drawing, that could perhaps be utilized in the class so that the child begins to develop an awareness of his/her role within the class. However, it is obvious that these skills must be kept in perspective and not allowed to dominate either that child's behaviour or the rest of the class.

13 Emphasize the importance of the child looking at you when he/she speaks and also when he/she listens.

14 Keep instructions simple and unambiguous. Bear in mind that the children may have little idea of what to focus on or what is relevant. Therefore they have great difficulty extracting information and using it meanfully.

15 Try and keep your language fairly concrete. Try and avoid metaphor, sarcasm that may not be understood, and too many colloquialisms.

16 Emphasize the importance of turn taking, and check that the child really understands what the concept of 'turns' means.

17 Reinforce any work on feelings so that the child begins to consider, not just the basic ones such as 'happy', 'cross' and 'sad', but 'fed up', 'tired', 'annoyed' and so on, and how other people feel.

18 Some children with an autistic spectrum disorder may appear aggressive towards other children. Sometimes this is because they want to be friends, but do not know how to go about it and use inappropriate strategies.

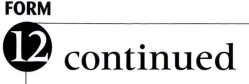

We have a number of books that we use specifically in the social skills groups and which the children enjoy. Some titles are listed below and may be of interest to you, especially if there are any opportunities for small-group work in school with learning support staff:

Aliki, *Feelings*, Macmillan Children's, London, 1994.

Aliki, *Manners*, Mammoth, 1994.

Aliki, *Communication*, Mammoth, 1995.

Goffe T (illus), *Bully For You*, Child's Play, Swindon, 1991.

Kelly A, *Talkabout*, Winslow, Bicester, 1996.

Moses B & Gordon M, *I Feel Angry,* Wayland, Hove, 1994.

Moses B & Gordon M, *I Feel Frightened,* Wayland, Hove, 1994.

Moses B & Gordon M, *I Feel Jealous,* Wayland, Hove, 1994.

Moses B & Gordon M, *I Feel Sad,* Wayland, Hove, 1994.

O'Neill C, *Relax,* illus. T Goffe, Child's Play, 1993.

Rinaldi W, *Social Use of Language Programme,* NFER Nelson, 1992.

Rinaldi W, *SULP Primary and Pre-school Teaching Pack,* (available from author: 18 Dorking Road, Chilworth, Surrey, GU4 8NR UK).

Appendix II
Useful addresses,
sources & resources

● United Kingdom

Advisory Centre for Education (ACE) Ltd
1b Aberdeen Studios
22 Highbury Grove
London N5 2DQ
Tel 0171-354 8318
Fax 0171-354 9069

AFASIC
347 Central Markets
London EC1A 9NH
Tel 0171-236 3632
Fax 0171-236 8115

The Association of Head Teachers of Adults and Children with Autism (AHTACA)
PO Box 2008
Maidenhead
Berkshire SL6 7FT

Autism Research Unit (NAS)
The School of Health Sciences
University of Sunderland
Sunderland SR2 7EE
Tel 0191-510 8922
Fax 0191-567 0420

The Centre for Social and Communication Disorders (NAS)
Elliot House
113 Masons Hill
Bromley
Kent BR2 9HT
Tel 0181-466 0098
Fax 0181-466 0118

Contact-a-Family
170 Tottenham Court Road
London W1P 0HA
Tel 0171-383 3555
Fax 0171-383 0259

Derbyshire Language Scheme
Market House
Market Place
Ripley
Derbyshire DE5 3BR
Tel 01773 748002

Dyslexia Institute
133 Gresham Road
Staines
Middlesex TW18 2AJ
Tel 01784 463851
Fax 01784 460747

Hanen UK/Ireland
9 Dungoyne Street
Maryhill
Glasgow G20 0BA
Scotland
Tel/Fax 0141 946 5433

ICAN
Barbican City Gate
1–3 Dufferin Street
London EC1Y 8NA
Tel 0171-374 4422
Fax 0171-374 2762

KIDS
(For Children with Special
Needs)
80 Wayneflete Square
London W10 6UD
Tel 0181-969 2817
Fax 0181-969 4550

Makaton
Makaton Vocabulary
Development Project
31 Firwood Drive
Camberley
Surrey GU15 3QD
Tel 01276 61390

Mencap
Mencap National Centre
123 Golden Lane
London EC1Y 0RT
Tel 0171-454 0454
Fax 0171-608 3254

**The National Autistic
Society (NAS)**
393 City Road
London EC1V 1NE
Tel 0171-833 2299
Fax 0171-833 9666

**The National Portage
Association**
127 Monk Dale
Yeovil
Somerset BA21 3JE
Tel/Fax 01935 471641
(Portage materials are published
by NFER-Nelson)

The Paget-Gorman Society
3 Gipsy Lane
Headington
Oxford OX3 7PT
Tel 01865 61908

**The Royal College of Speech
& Language Therapists**
7 Bath Place
Rivington Street
London EC2A 3DR
Tel 0171-613 3855
Fax 0171-613 3854

TEACCH (UK)
Mr K Lovett
Society for the Autistically
Handicapped (SFTAH)
199/201 Blandford Avenue
Kettering
Northants NN16 9AT
Tel/Fax 01536 523274

● **Canada**

Autism Society Canada
129 Yorkville Ave
Suite 202
Toronto M5R 1C4
Canada
Tel 1-416 922 0302
Fax 1-416 922 1032

The Geneva Centre
250 Davisville Ave
Suite 200
Toronto M4S 1HZ
Canada
Tel 1-416 322 7877
Fax 1-416 322 5894

The Hanen Program
252 Bloor St West
Suite 3-390
Toronto M5S 1V5
Canada
Tel 1-416 921 1073
Fax 1-416 921 1225

● United States of America

Autism Society of America
7910 Woodmount Ave
Suite 650
Bethesda
Maryland 20814-3015
USA
Tel 1-301 657 0881
Fax 1-301 657 0869

Future Horizons
422E Lamar #106
Arlington
Texas 76011
USA
Tel 1-817 277 0727
Fax 1-817 277 2270

TEACCH
Division TEACCH
310 Medical School Wing E
222H University of North
Carolina
Chapel Hill
NC 27514 USA
Tel 1-919 966 2174
Fax 1-919 966 4127

Useful books and equipment for intervention

We feel some ambivalence about suggesting specific books and equipment. Nothing dates a publication more than a list of recommendations that are either no longer obtainable or else have been superseded by more up-to-date and interesting material. However, it could also be argued that a sourcebook should specify these very things in order to provide readers with information which they would otherwise have to research for themselves. To accommodate both these positions, we are listing some items with the rider that they represent the *type* of equipment or book, rather than, necessarily, this or that particular item.

We would like to encourage users to browse regularly through catalogues, as well as local children's book and toy shops so that they refresh and update their equipment. Also special needs exhibitions are held regularly at different locations, and provide opportunities for seeing what products are available.

Because children with autism need so much reinforcement it is important to ensure that equipment is varied and interesting. It is not only the children who need variety: therapists and teachers can become repetitive and stale without the stimulation and challenge of something new. Sometimes it is a good idea to defer spending a budget until a group is under way, since the needs of particular children may influence purchasing choices.

Books

Aliki, *Feelings*, Macmillan Children's, London, 1994.

Aliki, *Manners*, Mammoth, 1994.

Aliki, *Communication*, Mammoth, 1995.

Children's Book Week Joke Book, Macmillan Children's, London, 1994.

Cumine V, Leach J & Stevenson G, *Asperger Syndrome: A Practical Guide for Teachers,* David Fulton, London, 1998.

Gray C et al, *The New Social Story Book*, Future Horizons, Arlington TX, 1994.

Hodgson L, *Visual Strategies for Improving Communication* Volume 1, Quirk Roberts, Michigan, 1995.

Kelly A, *Talkabout*, Winslow, Bicester, 1996.

Listening Skills — Key Stage 1, The Questions Publishing Company Ltd, Birmingham,

Listening Skills — Key Stage 2, The Questions Publishing Company Ltd, Birmingham,

Martin L, *Think It — Say It*, Communication Skill Builders, Tuscon AZ, 1990.

Moses B & Gordon M, *Your Emotions Series*, Wayland, Hove, 1993.
I Feel Sad;
I Feel Angry;
I Feel Jealous;
I Feel Frightened;
(Further titles from Wayland include *I'm Bored*, *I'm Lonely*, *I'm Worried*, *It's Not Fair*.)
O'Neill C, *Relax,* illus. T. Goffe, Child's Play, 1993.

Rinaldi W, *Social Use of Language Programme*, NFER-Nelson, Windsor, 1992.

Rinaldi W, *SULP Primary and Pre-school Teaching Pack* (available from author: 18 Dorking Road, Chilworth, Surrey GU4 8NR UK), 1994.

Rosen M, *Hairy Tales and Nursery Crimes,* Young Lions, London, 1987.

Schroeder A, *Socially Speaking*, LDA, Cambridge, 1996.

Goffe T (illus), *Bully For You,* Child's Play, Swindon, 1991.

Video

See What I Mean (obtainable from ICAN). This includes a range of emotions which are portrayed by actors without the use of words.

Equipment

For young children it is useful to acquire a small selection of fun toys and activities which will provide an incentive for turn taking: such things as a marble run, bubbles, slinkies, in fact anything which is engaging for a short time, and small enough to be handed over easily to the next child.

Many useful items of equipment are obtainable from special needs suppliers. Examples of these are listed below:

• United Kingdom

Learning Development Aids
Park Works
Norwich Road
Wisbech
Cambridgeshire PE13 2AE
*Publish a mail-order catalogue for
children with special needs*

NFER-Nelson
Darville House
2 Oxford Road East
Windsor
Berks SL4 1DF
Publishers of SULP *and*
Understanding Ambiguity

Rompa
Goyt Side Road
Chesterfield
Derbyshire S40 2BR
*Specialise in sensory equipment for
children with special needs*

Speechmark Publishing Ltd
8 Oxford Court
St James Road
Brackley
Northants NN13 7XY
www.speechmark.net
*Publishers of ColorCards, publications
and other resources for children and
adolescents with special needs*

• Australia

Modern Teaching Aids
26-28 Chard Road
Brookvale
NSW 2100
*Educational catalogue of resources
suitable for students with special
needs*

• Canada

Braut & Bouthillier
700 Avenue Beaumont
Montreal H3N 1V5
www.brautbouthillier.com
*Educational catalogue featuring
toys and many items for teachers
of children with special needs*

PsyCan Corp
Unit 12
120 West Beaver Creek Road
Richmond Hill
Ontario L4B 1L2
*Distributors of materials for
speech & language therapy*

• United States of America

S&S Worldwide
75 Mill Street
PO Box 513
Colchester
Connecticut 06415
Games and educational toys catalogues

The Speech Bin
1965 Twenty-fifth Avenue
Vero Beach
Florida 32960
*Mail-order catalogue with workbooks
and picture cards for speech &
language pathologists*

Super Duper Publications
PO Box 24997
Greenville
South Carolina 29616-2497
www.superduperinc.com
*Range of workbooks and games
for all children with special needs*

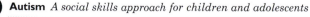

Bibliography

Aarons M & Gittens T, *The Autistic Continuum: An Assessment and Intervention Schedule*, NFER-Nelson, Windsor, 1992.

Aarons M & Gittens T, *The Handbook of Autism: A Guide for Parents and Professionals*, Routledge, London, 1992.

Aarons M & Gittens T, '"A Little Bit Autistic": An Overview of the Difficulties of Young Children at the Upper End of the Autistic Continuum', 1995. (Available from Autism Advisers, 8 Winscombe Crescent, London W5 1AZ.)

AHTACA, *The Special Curricular Needs of Autistic Children*, AHTACA, London, 1985. (Available from NAS, new edition pending.)

AHTACA, *The Special Curricular Needs of Autistic Children: Learning and Thinking Skills*, AHTACA, London, 1990. (Available from NAS.)

Bailey A, Phillips W & Rutter M, 'Autism: Towards an Integration of Clinical, Genetic, Neuropsychological and Neurobiological Perspectives', *Journal of Child Psychology and Psychiatry* 37 (1), 1996.

Baron-Cohen S, *Mindblindness: An Essay on Autism and Theory of Mind*, MIT Press, Cambridge MA, 1995.

Baron-Cohen S & Bolton P, *Autism: The Facts*, Oxford University Press, Oxford, 1993.

Baron-Cohen S, Allen J & Gillberg C, 'Can Autism be Detected at 18 Months? The Needle, the Haystack and the CHAT', *British Journal of Psychiatry* 161, 1992.

Baron-Cohen S, Tager-Flusberg H & Cohen D (eds), *Understanding Other Minds: Perspectives from Autism*, Oxford University Press, Oxford, 1993.

Biklen D, *Communication Unbound: How Facilitated Communication is Challenging Traditional Views of Autism and Ability/Disability*, Teachers College Press, New York, 1993.

Bishop D, 'Autism, Asperger's Syndrome and Semantic-Pragmatic Disorder: Where are the Boundaries?', *British Journal of Disorders of Communication* 24(2), 1989.

Cooper J, Moodley M & Reynell J, *Helping Language Development*, Edward Arnold, London, 1978.

Davies J, *Children with Autism: a booklet for brothers and sisters*, University of Nottingham, 1993. (Available from NAS.)

Davies J, *Able Autistic Children – Children with Asperger Syndrome: a booklet for brothers and sisters*, University of Nottingham, 1994. (Available from NAS.)

De Bono E, *Teach your Child How to Think*, Penguin, London, 1993.

Department of Education and Employment, *Excellence for all Children: Meeting Special Educational Needs*, The Stationery Office, London, 1997.

DiLavore C, Lord C & Rutter M, 'The Pre-Linguistic Autism Diagnostic Observation Schedule', *Journal of Autism and Developmental Disorder* 25(4), 1995.

Frith U, *Autism: Explaining the Enigma*, Blackwell, Oxford, 1989.

Frith U (ed.), *Autism and Asperger Syndrome*, Cambridge University Press, Cambridge, 1991.

Gagnon L, Mottron L & Joanette Y, 'Questioning the Validity of the Semantic–Pragmatic Syndrome Diagnosis', *Autism: The International Journal of Research and Practice* 1 (1), 1997.

Grandin T, *Thinking in Pictures and other reports from my life with autism*, Vintage, New York, 1996.

Happe F, *Autism: An Introduction to Psychological Theory*, UCL Press, London, 1994.

Howlin P, *Autism: Preparing for Adulthood*, Routledge, London, 1997.

Jordan R & Powell S, *Understanding and Teaching Children with Autism*, Wiley, Chichester, 1995.

Kanner L, 'Autistic Disturbances of Affective Contact', *Nervous Child* 2 (217), 1943.

King L, 'Sensory Integration: An Effective Approach to Therapy and Education', *Autism Research Review International* 5 (2), 1991.

Knowles W & Masidlover M, *Derbyshire Language Scheme*, Derbyshire County Council Education Psychology Service, Ripley, 1980.

Lovaas O, 'The UCLA Young Autism Model of Service Delivery' in **Maurice C (ed.)**, *Behavioural Intervention for Young Children with Autism*, Pro-Ed, Austin, 1996.

Ozonoff S, Strayer D, McMahon W & Filloux F, 'Executive Function Abilities in Autism: An Information Processing Approach', *Journal of Child Psychology and Psychiatry* 35, 1994.

Rapin I, 'Developmental Language Disorders: A Clinical Update', *Journal of Child Psychology and Psychiatry* 37 (6), 1996.

Rimland B & Edelson S, 'Brief Report: A Pilot Study of Auditory Integration Training in Autism', *Journal of Autism and Developmental Disorder* 25 (61).

Rinaldi W, *Social Use of Language Programme*, NFER-Nelson, Windsor, 1992.

Rinaldi W, *SULP Primary and Pre-school Teaching Pack*, 1994. (Available from author, 18 Dorking Road, Chilworth, Surrey, GU4 8NR, UK.)

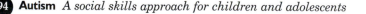

Rinaldi W, *Understanding Ambiguity: An Assessment of Pragmatic Meaning*, NFER-Nelson, Windsor, 1996.

Rinaldi W, *SULP Story Pack for Secondary School and College Students*, 1997. (Available from author, as above.)

Roberts J, 'Echolalia and Comprehension in Autistic Children', *Journal of Autism and Developmental Disorder* 19 (2), 1989.

Rustin L & Kuhr A, *Social Skills & The Speech Impaired*, Taylor & Francis, London, 1992.

Sacks O, *An Anthropologist on Mars*, Picador, London, 1995.

Schopler E & Mesibov G, *High Functioning Individuals with Autism*, Plenum, New York & London, 1992.

Spence S, *Social Skills Training: Enhancing Social Competence with Children and Adolescents*, NFER-Nelson, Windsor, 1995.

Tager-Flusberg H & Anderson M, 'The development of contingent discourse ability in autistic children', *Journal of Child Psychology and Psychiatry* 32 (7), 1991.

Treffert D, *Extraordinary People*, Bantam Press, London, 1989.

Williams D, *Nobody Nowhere*, Doubleday, London, 1992.

Williams D, *Somebody Somewhere*, Doubleday, London, 1994.

Williams D, *Autism: An Inside-Out Approach*, Jessica Kingsley Publications, London, 1996.

Wing L (ed.), *Aspects of Autism: Biological Research*, Gaskell/NAS, London, 1988.

Wing L, *The Autistic Spectrum: A Guide for Parents and Professionals*, Constable, London, 1996.

Wing L & Gould J, 'Severe Impairments of Social Interaction and Abnormalitites in Children: Epidemiology and classification', *Journal of Autism and Developmental Disorder* 9 (1), 1979.

Wolff S, *Loners: The Life Path of Unusual Children*, Routledge, London, 1995.

Index

adolescents *see* **older children and adolescent groups**
aggression 41–2
anxieties 42
appropriate behaviour 57–8, 64
Asperger Syndrome 2, 3
assertiveness skills 59
assessment 7–8
  anomalous behaviours 9
  birth history 8
  cognitive processes 10–12
  early social development 9
  language 12–13
  level of attention 9–10
  pre-school 25
  quality of play 10
  sensory dysfunction 10
attention 9–10, 22
attractive appearance 2–3, 9
autism
  continuum concept 2, 13
  as developmental disability 5–6, 8, 11–12
  as emotional disorder 3
  and learning disability 12
  phenotype 2, 7
  as social disability 1

babyhood 8–9, 22
Baron-Cohen, S. 5, 9, 23, 81
behaviours
  aggressive 41–2
  among peers 21
  anomalous 9
  appropriate 57–8, 64
  clinging 27
  disruptive 52–3
  positive 39
  repetitive and ritualistic 43
body language 47
books 31

central coherence, weak 5, 10–11, 15, 49, 51
CHAT *see* **Checklist for Autism in Toddlers (CHAT)**
Checklist for Autism in Toddlers (CHAT) 9, 23, 81
clinging behaviour 27
clinic-based social skills training 38, 63
cognitive abilities 23, 27, 56
  assessment 10–12
cognitive development 5, 10–11, 15, 49, 51, 55
  pyramid 26
communication *see* **language**
counselling 19

diagnosis 2–4
  classification systems vs intuition 14
  descriptive traits 15
  extension of criteria 7
  without support 23
disruptive behaviour 52–3

evaluation 64
  parental 77
  professional 78
  progress file 75–6
everyday routines 22–3
eye contact 22, 30

families
  autism features in 2, 7
  and emotional/behavioural problems 3, 42, 43
  negotiation within 58
  support of 18–19
  see also **parents**
feelings 46–7, 48
food allergies 33, 73
Frith, U. 5, 10

games 29–31
  adapting to reflect progress 48–9
  bath time 23
  question words 39
  sequencing and memory 51
  showing and identifying feelings 47
good sitting 29, 38–9
group leaders 65
group management issues 52–3
groups *see* **social skills training groups**

Hanen 18
home-based intervention programmes 18, 25

idioms 56
inappropriate behaviour *see* **appropriate behaviour**
independence, promotion of 59–61, 65
infant groups 37–9
  activities 40–1
  problems 41–3
  session plan 79
inference 56
islets of ability 4, 8
  expressive language 13

jokes 56–7
junior groups
  body language 47
  concept of manners 45, 46–7
  group management issues 52–3
  problems 47–8
  suggestions for activities 48–51

language
 abnormalities 4
 assessment 12–13
 conversation skills 39, 49–50, 56–7
 for older children 56–7
 question words 39
 and social impairments 4, 13
 Social Use of Language Programme
  (SULP) 5, 38–9, 55
 therapists 4, 12–13, 14, 19, 41
learning disability 12
 terminology 18
life skills 55
 exercises 60
listening skills 49

mainstream schools
 exchange visits 60–1
 social skills training groups 37–8, 63
 teachers' handout 83–5
 vs special schools 34–5
manners 45, 46–7, 48, 57
 showing sympathy and concern 58–9
manual sign systems 4, 39
mentalizing see theory of mind
metaphors 56
'miracle cures' 6, 67

National Autistic Society 8, 19, 25
negotiation skills 58
'news time' 49–50, 57
nursery rhymes 22
nursery school placement 21
 social skills gained from 27

older children and adolescent groups 55–6
 appropriate behaviour 57–8
 conversation exercises 56–7
 making choices 59–61
 role-play 58–9, 61, 64
other people, understanding 5, 10–11, 45, 49
'own space' 50

parents
 commitment 63, 66
 expectations 5–6, 12–13, 26, 64
 and growing up 59, 65
 information from 47, 49
 involvement in groups 65
 paperwork 72–4, 77, 80
 pre-school role 22–3, 25
 support of 23–5
 workshops 24–5, 73–4
 see also families
personal safety 61
photographs 22, 29, 51–2
physical contact 50
pictures
 illustrated stories 38
 in life skills exercises 60
 sequencing 11, 29, 51
play
 assessment 10
 free and routine 32
 lap 22
 see also games
play groups see nursery school placement
pointing 22, 23
Portage 18
pre-school activities 21–4
pre-school assessment 25
pre-school groups 26–9
 sessions 28–9
 suggested activities 29–31

referral 63, 71
remediation approaches 1, 3–4, 5
repetitive and ritualistic behaviours 5, 43
respite care facilities 19
Rinaldi, W. 6, 38, 55
role-play 48–9
 for older children 58–9, 61, 64
rote learning 12
SENCOs see Special Educational Needs
  Co-ordinators (SENCOs)
sensory dysfunction 3–4, 10
snack time 21–2, 30, 40
 and cooking 31
social impairments 2, 5, 15
 and language 4, 13
social skills training groups
 aims 26
 developmental approach 27
 duration of session 66
 human resources 65
 location 63
 paperwork 63–4, 71–85
 size 27
 video monitoring 64
 see also infant groups, junior groups,
  older children and adolescent groups,
  pre-school groups
Social Use of Language Programme (SULP)
  6, 38–9, 55
Special Educational Needs Co-ordinators
  (SENCOs) 44, 60, 82
special schools
 exchange visits 60–1
 social skills training groups 37
 vs mainstream schools 34–5
speech and language therapists 4, 12–13, 14,
  19, 41
spontaneity 55
Statement of Special Educational Needs 18,
  34–5, 37
stories 38, 47–8
SULP see Social Use of Language
  Programme (SULP)
teachers' handout 83–5
terminology 2, 17–18
theory of mind 5, 10, 11, 15, 49, 55
'time line' 28
timetables, visual 29
Triad of Social Impairments 2, 5, 13, 15
turn-taking
 activities 31, 49–50, 59
 stories 38
understanding
 concept of 'other people' 5, 10–11, 45, 49
 language 13
 'meaningfulness' 5, 10–11
 reasons for group attendance 52
variability 2
 developmental aspects 8
 fluctuations of mood 42
 individual uniqueness 4, 67
 low- and high-functioning children 12
video monitoring 64
visual aids see photographs, pictures,
  timetables
white lies 11, 58
Wing, L. 2, 5

Also available from Speechmark ...

We publish and distribute a wide range of resources for speech & language and social skills. Listed below are just a few of these – a full catalogue is available on request.

Talkabout
Alex Kelly

Providing practioners with a comprehensive framework for the development of social communication skills, this photocopiable manual can be used with children, adolesecents and adults.

Talkabout Activities
Alex Kelly

Containing 225 group activities, this excellent resource is aimed primarily at people familiar with *Talkabout*, although it can be used by anyone running social skills groups and will complement other social-skills training programmes.

Working with Pragmatics
Lucie Anderson-Wood & Benita Rae-Smith

Contains practical pragmatic teaching activities to develop communication skills. Offers an opportunity to explore this subject with confidence and to plan intervention programmes for effective management. Photocopiable assessment forms are included.

The Social Skills Handbook
Sue Hutchings, Jayne Comins & Judy Offiler

A range of useful and adaptable ideas and activities can be found in this practical guide which has been specifically designed for anyone running social skills groups. All activities are designed to be photocopied.

Social Skills Programmes: An Integrated Approach from Early Years to Adolescence
Maureen Aarons & Tessa Gittens

Following on from *Autism*, this new publication contains detailed photocopiable sesson plans for early years, infants, juniors and adolescents.

Writing & Developing Social Stories: Practical Interventions in Autism
Caroline Smith

This practical resource provides an introduction to the theory and practice of writing social stories. In addition, there are examples of successful stories to use as guides, as well as information and photocopiable resources for delivering training on the use of social stories.

Semantic-Pragmatic Language Disorder
Charlotte Firth & Katherine Venkatesh

Designed to fill the need for materials that provide a practical framework to identify, treat and manage Semantic-Pragmatic disorder in children. It has grown out of the authors' day-to-day experiences of working with these children and their families, and the therapy ideas offered are a selection of the best activities that have proved effective in everyday use.

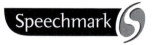
Speechmark